The Doctors Who Give No Medicine

The Science and Results
of
Upper Cervical Spinal Care

Dr Jeffrey Hannah DC, BSc

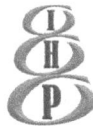

International Health Publishing
Carrollton, Texas, USA

INTERNATIONAL HEALTH PUBLISHING
Since February 2008
Publishing Group Affirming Truth & Innate Wisdom

For information about special discounts for bulk purchase, please contact International Health Publishing at writer@InternationalHealthPublishing.com.

International Health Publishing can bring authors to your live events. To book an event contact writer@InternationalHealthPublishing.com, or visit our website: www.InternationalHealthPublishing.com.

The Doctors Who Give No Medicine
The science and results of upper cervical spinal care

Dr Jeffrey Hannah DC
www.atlashealth.com.au

ISBN-13 978-0-9857956-4-1

E-Pub ISBN-13 978-0-9857956-5-8

Library of Congress Control Number: 2013931157

SAN   856-6925

The Doctors Who Give No Medicine

The Science and Results
of
Upper Cervical Spinal Care

Dr Jeffrey Hannah DC

"For my parents David and Joan,
and for my wife Natalie,
whose faith, inspiration and love
have made this book possible."

Contents

Introduction

*What lies behind us and what lies before us are
small matters compared to what lies within us.
And when we bring what is within us out into
the world, miracles happen.*

Ralph Waldo Emerson

"Hi Jeffrey. It's Dad. I don't know when you'll get this message, but I need you to come to the clinic to take an emergency upper cervical x-ray series. Call me back when you can. Bye."

It was 10:00am on an early autumn day, and I had just returned from a casual morning run when I discovered this message on my mobile phone.

It was also the end of my clinical residency at Palmer College in Davenport, Iowa. After seven years of intensive study, I had finished all of my graduation requirements, and I was trying to enjoy some well-earned relaxation time. Basically, I was aiming to do as little as possible until the graduation ceremony just two weeks away.

My dad, Dr Hannah was one of the clinic staff doctors, who supervised the student interns. Although I didn't do my internship directly under him, I worked with many of his patients and still tried to pick his brain for as much information as possible.

As part of my internship, I also worked as a radiology technician, aka "blue coat." Basically I was a junior supervisor, who assisted the other interns when they needed to take x-rays. One of the perks of the job was that you could complete all your x-ray requirements easily within just a few weeks. Most other interns would struggle for months!

Dad knows that I finished my x-ray numbers a year ago. I thought. Why does he need me? Why not find another intern, who still needs their numbers? Besides, what is an emergency upper cervical x-ray series?

I had never heard of such a thing! Surely I must have misheard him. I replayed the message.

"Hi Jeffrey. It's Dad. I don't know when you'll get this message, but I need you to come to the clinic to take an emergency upper cervical x-ray series. Call me back when you can. Bye."

Upper Cervical referred to an advanced group of techniques taught at Palmer, two of which I had studied in my previous term. Although I was not yet an expert, my experience as a blue coat gave me a confidence that few other interns possessed: that is, I felt comfortable taking and analyzing the unique type of x-rays, which are required for Upper Cervical work.

In fact, Dr Hannah would intentionally schedule his interns to take their x-rays during my radiology shifts. That way I could make sure that all the x-rays that he needed were taken properly.

Strangely, this was the first time that he had ever asked for help outside of my normal hours.

It seemed even stranger that he was asking for "and emergency upper cervical x-ray series." I had always believed that Upper Cervical treatment was only for chronic problems. Indeed, every upper cervical patient I had seen at Palmer had a chronic problem such as headaches, tingling in the fingers or jaw-related symptoms.

But never acute symptoms! Adding to my confusion, we only took emergency x-rays for real nasty problems like a dislocated joint or a fractured bone.

What is an emergency upper cervical x-ray series? I thought again. What is going on?

I returned my dad's call but only got through to one of his interns. "I don't know where Dr Hannah is, but he did say he still wants you to come to the clinic if you can."

"... I'll be right there," I responded after a momentary hesitation. So much for my lazy morning!

The clinic was less than a two-minute trot across the street, but I still had to cleanup from my run. Halfway though my shower, I realised I had a small but significant problem: I didn't have my clinic uniform!

It was strict Palmer policy that no intern was to work, let alone enter the clinic without wearing the proper attire. I had no dress shirt, no dress pants, no shoes, no tie and no white doctor's coat.

All I had was a t-shirt, jean shorts, and a pair of dirty runners.

Well, if this is truly an emergency, they won't care what I'm wearing.

Although I was finished with clinic, I still didn't want a reprimand from the disciplinary committee. I slipped through the rear entrance of the clinic and sneaked into Dr Hannah's office.

The intern to whom I'd spoken on the phone had still not seen my dad, but he did inform me that Dr White (one of the other staff doctors) was on duty and looking for me.

No sooner did I step out of the office, he found me. Although I did not dress the part, I did my best to maintain my professionalism. "Dr White, have you seen Dr Hannah?"

In a calm yet urgent tone, he responded, "No, but your dad's been waiting for you. We've got a little situation on our hands."

Dr White led me to a treatment room in the farthest, quietest corner of the clinic, peeked his head inside and spoke softly, "How's it going?"

I could not see anything inside the room. It was completely black. I could only hear a small muffled response.

"Hang in there. We're just about ready to go." Dr White spoke again.

As Dr White closed the door, he turned to me with eyes wide and sighed deeply.

"Dr White," I asked finally, "what is going on?"

I never imagined that inside that black room I would experience something that would so completely change my perspective on chiropractic and on health.

Before I entered that black room, I knew that chiropractic worked. However, all I knew was the type of chiropractic that most people know: general spinal manipulation.

I never knew that there was another way. And I never knew about the amazing results that it could achieve.

I never knew about Upper Cervical care.

The brain controls all messages to every cell in the entire body, including messages of health and healing.

The upper cervical spine—the atlas and the axis—directly affects the spinal cord and the brainstem, which is the control centre of the brain.

If the upper cervical spine is not aligned, the brain is not able to communicate properly with the rest of the body. As a direct consequence, health problems will begin to appear.

Upper Cervical is a specialist approach to chiropractic that corrects the misalignment of the atlas and axis, thereby restoring the health and optimal wellbeing of the body.

If these four sentences make sense to you, you do not need to read any further into this book. That is the essence of Upper Cervical care. However, if you want to discover its deeper power, please read onward. I have written this book for you.

As a disclaimer, I must add that the information contained in this book is for educational purposes only and not intended to treat or diagnose any person with any condition. Moreover, for all the incredible stories that you will read, remember that Upper Cervical is not a cure-all for all humanity's ailments.

I will still declare here-and-now that any person who receives proper Upper Cervical care has a much better chance to recover from almost any ailment if just given the chance.

If you have been suffering, looking for answers, or just feeling lost, I hope that the following chapters and stories will invigorate your spirit. I hope that you will better understand the awesome power that is within you; and I hope that you will take action to live the full and energetic life that you desire.

Dr Jeffrey Hannah
Upper Cervical Chiropractor

CHAPTER 1

Anatomy 101

*I am a doctor. My job is simple. All I have to do is
know everything about every disease
in the known universe.*

Author Unknown

Life requires the harmonious balance of the body, the mind
and the spirit.

Anything that disrupts this balance has the potential to affect
our health.

Cigarettes, synthetic food, skin products, mobile phones,
traffic jams, the six o'clock news, sedentary jobs, extreme sports
or any other form of stress you can imagine: all these things
affect our bodies and ultimately our health.

There is not one solution to the many problems that exist in the world. Fortunately, there is an internal life force that resides within each of us, which heals us and sustains our wellbeing.

Some call this force homeostasis, or the natural healing mechanisms of the body. Others call it innate intelligence or the Qi (chi). Whatever you choose to call it, it exists. Science and medicine still struggle to demonstrate its existence empirically, but with absolute certainty it exists just the same.

This critical centre from which this life force flows, giving life to your body is located just two-finger widths below the base of your skull. It is this area that is known as the upper cervical spine.

———————

Before we examine what Upper Cervical care does and how it works, it will help if we cover a few basics and introduce the players involved:

- The atlas
- The axis
- The brain and
- The nervous system, which controls everything in the body.

You do not need to be an expert in neuroanatomy, in order to understand Upper Cervical care. Better yet, you do not need to know everything about every disease in the known universe.

As a friendly warning, the first section of this book contains some scientific trivia and a few numbers. If you are not inclined toward these types of details, read only the sentences written in a boldface font to get the core messages. Then skip ahead to the end of each chapter where you will find the executive summary.

It is my hope that you will enjoy the entirety of this book and appreciate all the intricate details that are involved with Upper Cervical Care. Moreover, I think that you will be pleasantly surprised to discover that despite the technical details, the principles of Upper Cervical care are actually pretty simple.

Shall we begin?

Atlas and Axis

Atlas.   According to Greek mythology, following the war between the Olympian gods and the Titans, Zeus condemned Atlas to support the sky and heavens above the earth.   In modern and classic sculpture, Atlas is seen holding the weight of the world upon his shoulders.

The atlas (also known as C1) is also the name of the first cervical vertebra in the neck (Figure 1.1).   It weighs only 50 grams but supports the entire weight of your head, which is approximately 4.0 - 5.0 kilograms (8-10 pounds). [i] [ii]

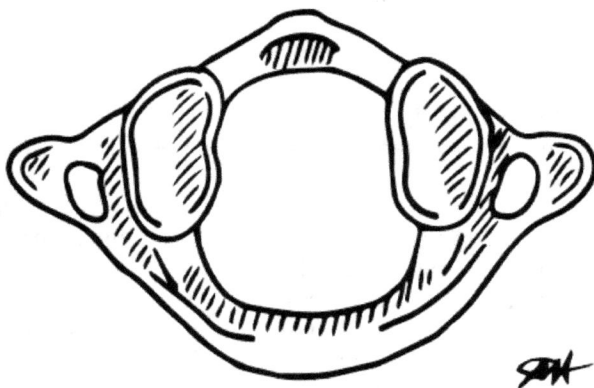

Figure 1.1 Atlas Vertebra

Imagine a bowling ball sitting on top of a small mobile phone. It is quite a disproportionate difference when you think of it that way! Nevertheless that is exactly how your body is constructed.

Just as Atlas holds the weight of the world on his shoulders, so too does your atlas; it hold your world (your head).

As you can see in Figure 1.1, the atlas is ring-shaped. The back two-thirds of the ring (bottom) is the sitting place of the brainstem, which connects the brain with the spinal cord. The front third of the inner ring (top) pivots around the second vertebra in the neck (also known as C2). It is because of this pivoting action that the C2 vertebra has its own unique name: the axis (Figure 1.2).

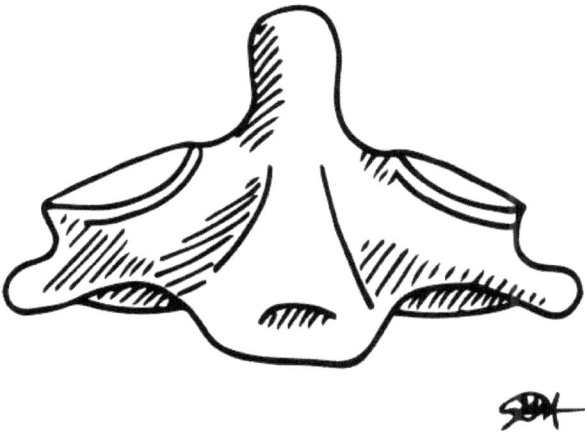

Figure 1.2 Axis Vertebra

The atlas is suspended between the head and the axis by sensitive muscles and ligaments. It is a small but critical point to make: the atlas is not held by any rigid or interlocking joint. This arrangement allows for a tremendous amount of motion between C1 and C2. Almost half of all your total neck movement—50% of the up-and-down and 50% of the total rotational movement—occurs in the upper cervical spine. [iii]

The atlas pivots around the axis, all the while supporting the weight of your head.

All other vertebrae from C3 to the sacrum (aka tailbone) contain interlocking joints that provide great stability but offer limited movement.

Think of your shoulder. You are probably able to move it almost 360 degrees in any direction. Compare that to your elbow joint, which only moves up-and-down. In terms of mobility, that is the difference between the upper cervical spine and the rest of the vertebral column.

The tradeoff is as follows: the more stability (bony locks), the less movement: but the more movement, the less stability. The importance of this arrangement shall be made clear shortly and then elaborated in subsequent chapters.

For the interim, let it suffice so say that the upper cervical spine is truly, "the most complex joints of the axial skeleton, both anatomically and kinematically." [iv]

———————————

Ideally, your head, atlas and axis are aligned perfectly straight relative to one another when your neck is in a neutral position: that is, the position that you believe is straight.

Of course, moving your head and neck changes this alignment. The atlas tilts forward and backward, side-to-side, and rotates left and right. When you return your head to a neutral position, the atlas should also return to its proper position.

The problem is that the atlas does not always return to its proper position.

If for some reason the atlas is knocked out of its normal alignment and cannot return to the neutral position, it creates an imbalance of the head and neck. Consequently, it is this imbalance that has the potential to cause major health problems elsewhere in the body.

We will see what causes a misalignment and what problems

may occur as a result in later chapters. For now, let's consider another very important part of the body: your central nervous system.

Subluxation

Subluxation is the traditional term used by chiropractors to describe a vertebral misalignment causing neurological interference. The term is an oft-debated, contentious issue among chiropractors and medical health professionals.

On one side, medical radiologists, orthopaedic specialists and surgeons use the word to describe a partial joint dislocation that has moved beyond its normal range of motion.

On the other side, chiropractors use the word to describe the abnormal fixation of a spinal vertebra within its normal range of motion that causes neurological dysfunction and biomechanical changes elsewhere in the body.

I must make it clear that there is a major difference between a chiropractic subluxation and a simple joint misalignment.

However, to minimise confusion for lay people who may be hearing of Upper Cervical care for the very first time, I will use the terms "subluxation" and "misalignment" interchangeably.

Where the word "subluxation" appears, it will be according to the chiropractic definition.

CHAPTER 2

Neurology 101

Get the big idea. All else follows.

Dr BJ Palmer

———————————

Your brain is an electrical generator. It is a battery that receives and gives rise to the energetic forces that flow through your body via your nervous system (Figure 2.1).

Imagine a powerful supercomputer connected to a high-speed Internet cable. Inside that cable are thousands of wires that connect to other smaller computers. That is how the nervous system is constructed. The supercomputer is your brain. The huge cables are your brainstem. Your spinal cord and nerves are the individual wires that ultimately connect to all the muscles, organs and tissues in your body.

In short, your nervous system is a communication network that connects your brain to every single cell in your body. It coordinates every sensation, emotion, movement and function that goes on in your body, including your health and ability to heal.

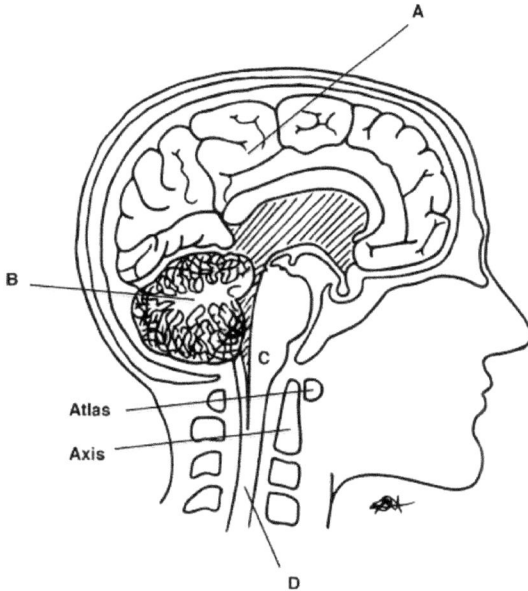

Figure 2.1 The Nervous System.
A. Cerebral Cortex. B. Cerebellum. C. Brainstem. D. Spinal Cord.

A functional nerve cell or neuron is capable of sending an electrical impulse at 275 kilometers (170 miles) per hour. [v] The same neuron is also capable of receiving 1000 other such impulses per second. It is estimated that there are 100 billion neurons in an adult human brain. Experts believe that the total computing capacity of the human brain is 400 billion bits of information per second. [vi vii]

Unless you are so inclined, there is no need to memorize these numbers. The take-home message is that the ability of your nervous system to send and receive information is so huge that I cannot even begin to describe it!

Even the fastest supercomputer in the world still cannot do the things that your body does every second of every day.

Of the 100 billion neurons in your brain, only 20 billion are located in the cerebral cortex (2.1a). [viii] The cerebral cortex is the upper part of your brain that coordinates the higher functions of human life: feeling (e.g., temperature and pain reception), special sensation (seeing and hearing), movement, learning, emotional processing and conscious awareness.

Amazing as those functions are, that means that 80 billion neurons—80% of all the neurons in your brain—are responsible for the primal, unconscious functions of life.

Of the 400 billion nerve impulses that our brain processes each second, we are only ever aware of about 2000 of them. [ix] That leaves 399,999,998,000 impulses per second that occur without our awareness.

In other words, 99.9999995% of all the neural messages that occur within your brains are completely unconscious.

Of the 80 billion neurons involved with unconscious processing, 60 billion are located within the cerebellum (2.1b).

The cerebellum is the cauliflower-shaped portion of the brain that coordinates all the signals about your body position, balance and internal awareness. Collectively, these internal feedback processes are known as proprioception

Close your eyes. Using your left hand, try to touch your nose. This is an example of proprioception. The information that your cerebellum processes allows you to do this action without poking yourself in the eye.

That is the awesome responsibility of your cerebellum: it is the primary processing centre that coordinates all the internal feedback messages that occur within your bodies so that you able to move like a human being.

Proprioception is internal body reception, and it is just as important as external body reception (e.g., sight, taste, touch, etc). Whether you are riding a bicycle, writing a letter, or doing any type of movement that requires skill, balance or fine motor coordination, proprioceptive messages are continuously streaming to and from your cerebellum.

If you take a moment to really think about it, you will realise that proprioception is involved with everything that you do! And it all happens without your conscious awareness.

———————————

The remaining 20 billion neurons involved with unconscious processing are located in the brainstem (2.1c). The brainstem is the lower core of the brain that coordinates the automatic processes of life: circulation, digestion, breathing, alertness, wakefulness and healing to name just a few.

Do you need to consciously think about your heart so that it maintains its proper rhythm? Or so that food moves properly though the 9.15m of your digestive system? Or so that your blood clots at the site of an open wound but not anywhere else?

These are the many processes of the brainstem. The brainstem is also the central hub where all information entering and exiting the brain passes. Known as the reticular formation, this structure acts like a filter or switchboard to relay signals to other locations within the brain.

The brainstem is the command centre that coordinates all messages between your brain and your body.

As a final word on basic neuroanatomy, there is one more important structure that deserves consideration: your spinal cord (2.1d). We will look at the spinal cord in greater detail in later chapters.

For now, the only thing you need to remember is the following sentence: the spinal cord is the communication conduit between your brain (cortex, cerebellum and brainstem) and the rest of your body.

Neuroanatomy 201

The human body is a marvel of engineering far more advanced than any supercomputer or artificial intelligence that mankind has yet created.

To illustrate that complexity, imagine that your brain generates a thought to wiggle your big toe. The thought actually involves thousands of impulses from the cerebral cortex and cerebellum, which filter into your brainstem. Your brainstem interprets these signals and then forwards the message to your spinal cord. The message is then sent down the correct neural pathway (wire) until it arrives at its destination: your big toe.

Sounds simple? However, multiply this simple example to include the 400 billion impulses occurring within your brain each second. Then multiply that number by the total number of seconds, hours, and years of your life.

Not so simple anymore, is it? Nevertheless, that is the amazing nature of your central nervous system. Hopefully it is clear that the capacity of your brain to receive, send and process information is beyond practical measure.

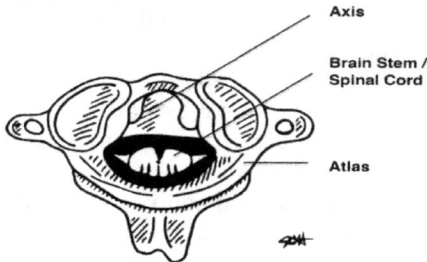

Figure 2.2 The Atlas, the Axis and the Spinal Cord.

For all the complex things described in this chapter about the atlas, the axis and the brain, there is really only one thing that you have to know in order to understand Upper Cervical care:

Your spinal cord passes directly through the top two vertebrae in your neck—the atlas and the axis. Therefore, any misalignment of those upper cervical vertebrae has the potential to affect transmission of signals between your brain and the rest of your nervous system and thus affect the function of your entire body.

That is the core principle of Upper Cervical care. For the all the complex structures that are involved, it is simple and makes a lot of sense.

As simple as this principle is, it did not come easily to me when I was studying chiropractic. None of the material was terribly difficult, but it was the sheer volume that overwhelmed me.

Chiropractic university is like opening your mouth to a fire hydrant and then trying to swallow as much water as possible. By the time you graduate, you are expected to have mastered 540 hours of anatomy, 320 hours of neurology, 360 hours of x-ray and 630 hours of medical diagnosis. And all that comes before 900 hours of your clinical residency. [x]

Alas, for all my hours in the library and clinic, there was nothing that prepared me for what I was about to see and experience in that dark room. Although I could recite a textbook full of facts about on upper cervical neuroanatomy and how the body heals itself, none of it was real.

In the next 90 minutes of my life, that was all about to change.

CHAPTER 3

Communication Gateway

Nature needs no help, just no interference.

Dr BJ Palmer

———————

"Oh good. You're here."

Dr Hannah appeared with a couple of students beside him. The first person was Kevin, a student still in his first year at Palmer but already a frequent clinic visitor with a strong interest in Upper Cervical care.

The second student I did not recognize. He would introduce himself later as Rob, one of Dr White's interns and a clinic rookie with very little knowledge of Upper Cervical care.

"Dr Hannah, what is going on?"

"Have you talked to Louise in radiology yet?" my dad asked.

Alas, he wasn't listening to me.

"No. Dad, what is going on?" I inquired more forcefully. This time, I did manage to get through to him.

"Let's go in here." He answered pointing toward an empty treatment room.

"I'll cover your students for the meantime," Dr White said to my dad. Clinic life would have to proceed as normal for the other patients and interns on duty that morning. With Dr White covering for him, that would be one less thing for my dad to worry about!

"Thank you," Dr Hannah replied.

That was the last I saw of Dr White that morning.

My dad motioned for Kevin, Rob and myself to follow him into the room. He closed the door, sighed and then proceeded to explain the situation.

"His name is Joe. Kevin brought him in about an hour ago. Basically he's having migraines and experiencing muscle weakness all throughout his body."

"What?" I interrupted, "What happened to him?"

Kevin continued the story. "He was at the student clinic last Friday, and they were working on his neck. Joe is one of my housemates, and when he got home he said he felt dizzy and was having trouble standing. He's been getting worse all weekend."

"Has he been to the hospital?"

"On Saturday. They did a CT, MRI and everything but sent him home yesterday."

"They what?!" I exclaimed.

"They said everything was okay and that they couldn't find anything wrong with him."

"He says he's seeing triple," my dad continued. "Not just double—triple! When he opens his eyes, he says his whole world gets blurry and starts to spin. It's been making him real sick. Plus he can't walk, let alone stand on his own. Kevin practically had to carry him in this morning. That's why he's lying down in the other room with the lights off."

I could not believe the story they were telling me. In my mind, there was only one thing I could think of that would explain Joe's symptoms.

My god! He's had a stroke!

"So what do you think it is?" I asked my dad fearfully.

"I know what you're thinking," he replied, "I don't think it's a stroke. Dr White also had a look at him, and he thinks the same thing."

"Are you sure?" I challenged.

It has long been my characteristic to challenge authority. This time, I was challenging the expert opinions of two chiropractic specialists with a combined 50 years of clinical experience. In hindsight, it seems so incredibly absurd!

"It doesn't fit," my dad responded. "Yes, he has the one- sided muscle weakness, but it's not in his eyes like it would be if he was having a stroke. Dr White did a complete neurological examination and thinks the problem is coming from somewhere in his upper neck. Dr White and I have talked about it, and we both think that we should try to adjust him with Upper Cervical."

"Are you sure?" I challenged again.

"No I'm not," my dad replied. "But he's already been to the hospital. They won't do anything. So what else can we do?"

The room fell into ominous silence.

I could hear the voices of my classroom instructors echoing in my head. Send him back to the hospital. He's having a stroke!

However, Dr Hannah did have a good point.

Joe had already been to the hospital. They had already performed all their tests, which would have shown clearly if he had suffered a stroke.

They found nothing, and they sent him home without any answers.

So what else can we do? My dad's words also echoed in my head—and fortunately his voice was louder and clearer than all the others.

What could it be if not a stroke? I thought to myself. I have no reason to doubt what Kevin and my dad have said. I'm sure Dr White would have performed dozens of tests I've never heard of. Still, even if his neck is out of alignment, how would an Upper Cervical treatment undo that amount of damage?

As if sensing my angst, my dad said the one thing that he knew would make my decision easier.

"You should see him for yourself."

━━━━━━━━━━━━━━━━

Imagine that you have an electrical problem in your home. For example, the power is not working in one bedroom. You contact an electrician, who traces the problem to a faulty wire near the switchboard. The electrician fixes the problem; and then like magic, the power comes back on in the bedroom.

Similarly, imagine that you have an electrical-type of problem in your body. For example, you are experiencing headaches. You contact an Upper Cervical doctor, who traces the problem to an inflamed nerve near the base of your skull. The doctor corrects the problem; and then like magic, the headache disappears.

With a basic understanding of the atlas, axis, the brain and the nervous system behind us, it is time to examine how the anatomy and neurology are connected. In this chapter, we will examine how a subluxation affects the spinal cord and can cause all sorts of problems.

The interesting thing is that as numerous as Joe's problems were, they are only the tip of the iceberg.

━━━━━━━━━━━━━━━━

The Spinal Cord

The spinal cord is the information superhighway of the nervous system (Figure 3.1). It is tethered onto the inner ring of the atlas with pieces of tissue shaped like tiny shark teeth called dentate ligaments.

Dentate ligaments are also present all the way from C2 to the tailbone. However, they are not nearly as short or thick as they are at the level of the atlas.

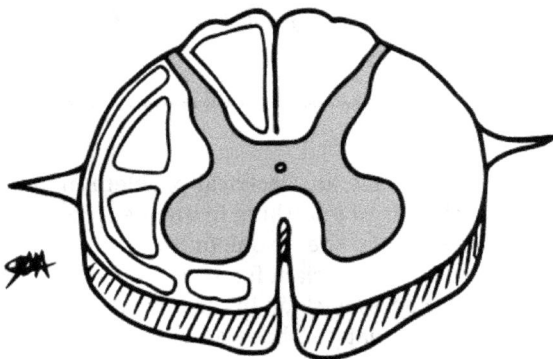

Figure 3.1 The Spinal Cord in Cross Section.

Imagine that you are holding a piece of string. First, picture you hold the string loosely and allow it to sag. Although the string is fixed on both ends, there is no tension. That is the way that dentate ligaments support the spinal cord below C2.

Next, imagine that you are hold the string tightly so that it is pulled taut—not too tight, but just so that there is a small amount of tension in the string. That is the way the dentate ligaments hold the spinal cord at the level of C1.

Now, hold the string taut just as you did before, but this time start pulling your hands apart. The tension in the string increases dramatically. It is in this same way that the atlas exerts tension on the spinal cord when it is misaligned.

Think of a radio. The dial must be tuned to the exact frequency in order to receive the clearest signal—otherwise the static or interference distorts the clarity of the messages.

In a similar manner, an atlas subluxation imparts tension through the dentate ligaments, which corrupts the clarity of messages transmitted along the spinal cord (Figure 3.2 and 3.3).

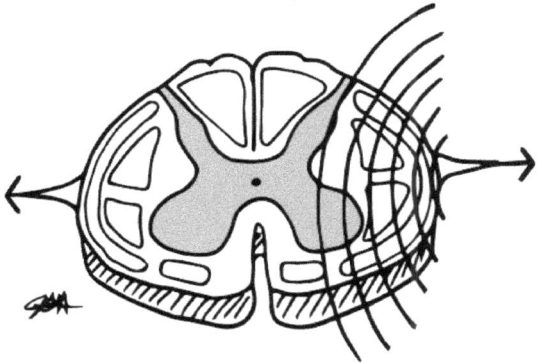

Figure 3.2 Spinal Cord Tension Caused by Pulling Stress.

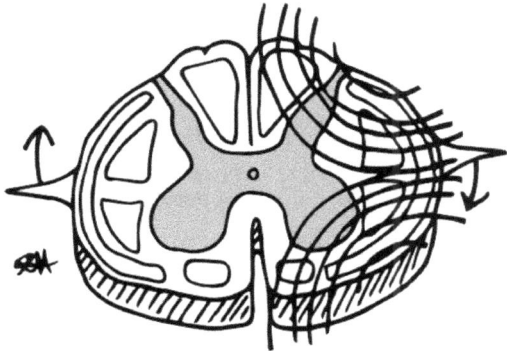

Figure 3.3 Spinal Cord Tension Caused by Rotational Stress.

If you twist your head for a couple of minutes, it usually does not cause any problems aside from a sore neck. However, if your atlas is knocked out of alignment and cannot return to the neutral position, the tension that accumulates in your muscles and in your spinal cord may become very significant as we will see in the next chapter.

CHAPTER 4

Communication Breakdown

Look well to the spine for the cause of disease.

Hippocrates

Like an electrical circuit, there is a fixed structural order of the wires within your spinal cord (Figure 4.1). When we consider that arrangement, we can see the exact types of problems that are possible from an upper cervical subluxation.

The dark sections of the spinal cord are groups of neurons, which are like mini switchboards within the nervous system. As a general rule, motor neurons (4.1a) send messages of movement to the muscles controlled by the C1 and C2 nerves. Motor neurons control the small suboccipital muscles that allow the atlas and axis to move. These neurons also control muscles on the front of the neck, the inner ear, and the powerful muscles that move the jaw.

Sensory neurons (4.1b) receive sensory feedback from all the internal and external receptors in the upper neck. Sensory neurons also receive feedback from the muscles and ligaments that support the atlas and axis. In addition, sensory neurons receive information from muscles along the front of the neck and from the trapezius (a broad muscle that extends across the back of the neck, the shoulders and wraps all the way to the middle back).

Dentate Ligaments

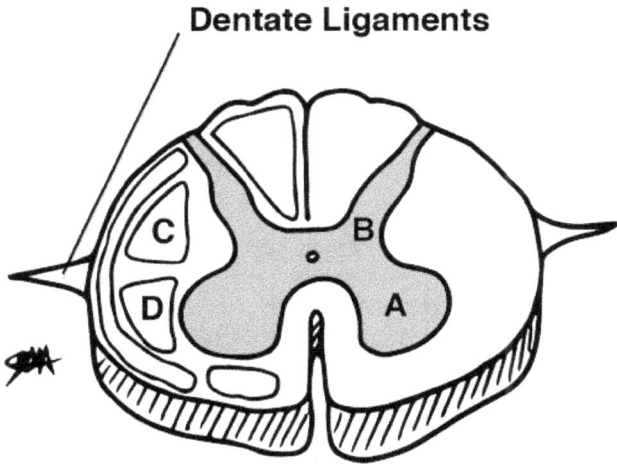

Figure 4.1 Groups of Wires within the Spinal Cord.
A. Motor Neurons. B. Sensory Neurons.
C. Corticospinal Tract. D. Spinothalamic Tract

There is also a special grouping of neurons in the upper cervical spine that receives sensory feedback from the Trigeminal Nerve, the 5th cranial nerve that conveys all sensory information from the head, the face and the jaw.

Spinal tension caused by a subluxation may corrupt the motor and sensory feedback mechanisms associated with that area of the body.

As a direct result, a person may suffer tightness or spastic muscles in the neck, shoulders, upper back, chest or jaw causing chronic soreness and fatigue.

You may suffer tension or sinus headaches, [xi xii xiii xiv] migraines, nausea, vomiting, or fainting spells. [xv xvi xvii]

You may also suffer suboccipital neuralgia, which is burning pain across the back of the head; or even trigeminal neuralgia, which is intense stabbing pain across the face. [xviii xix xx xxi xxii]

Trigeminal neuralgia is also known as "the suicide disease" and is universally regarded as the most painful condition known to medical science ranking above kidney stones, shingles and even childbirth.

The white sections of the spinal cord are tracts. Like telephone wires, they are the pathways that relay messages between the brain and the body. For our purposes, we will consider five major tracts: the corticospinal tracts, the spinothalamic tracts, the dorsal columns, the spinocerebellar tracts and the reticulospinal tracts.

The corticospinal tract (4.1c) is the motor pathway. It transmits signals from the motor cortex of the brain and brainstem to the neurons that control muscle function. They communicate messages of movement.

The spinothalamic tract (4.1d) is the sensory pathway. It transmits signals from sensory receptors throughout the body to a relay centre (the thalamus), which filters those signals to the sensory cortex of the brain. They communicate messages of temperature, pressure, movement and nociception, which are interpreted in the brain as pain.

With motor and sensory neurons (4.1a and 4.1b), spinal tension affects the cells in the upper neck only. However, spinal tension affecting the tracts adds a different dynamic to the problem. Distortion of the messages traveling along the communication pathways may create muscle tension, pain or other abnormal sensations anywhere in the body.

The result is that you may suffer shooting pains into the arms and hands, [xxiii] [xxiv] stabbing pains between the shoulders and ribs, lower back pain, [xxv] [xxvi] [xxvii] [xxviii] [xxix] [xxx] or even pain and tingling-sensations in the hands and feet. [xxxi] [xxxii] [xxxiii]

———————————

Case Report: Diabetic Neuropathy

James was referred to my office with acute lower back pain. Still working as a furniture removalist in his 60s, it was no surprise to me that he was having problems!

James was also a type II diabetic. Although his blood sugar levels were not dangerously high, his lifestyle choices over the course of many years left him with a number of issues including diabetic neuropathy, which is a constant tingling or numbness in his fingers and toes.

After an x-ray and then the initial treatment, James reported that his back was still pretty sore. On a positive note, he did notice that is was a little easier to lean forward.

"Just from that?" he asked with a puzzled expression, pointing to the spot where I had adjusted his neck.

"Just from that." I affirmed.

James returned two days later with more good news. He described that the sharp sensation in his lower back was completely gone, and that the only thing left was a bit of muscle soreness.

James added that something strange happened as well. He said that for the first day after I adjusted him, the tingling in his fingers and toes had disappeared completely.

The symptoms had since returned, but for the first time in about 10 years James could actually feel his feet!

Over the next month with successive adjustments, we managed to reduce the tingling in James's feet for almost a whole week at a time. Unfortunately, James's job required him to work long irregular hours, and we were not able to pursue a proper course of treatment thereafter.

I have since seen several more people who have reported similar tingling sensations in their fingers and toes, and many of them have also responded extremely well with Upper Cervical care.

I had assumed that the tingling in James's legs was due to his diabetes. In hindsight, it appears that I assumed wrong. It goes to show that a symptom—even if you think it is related to something else—may just be another manifestation of an Upper Cervical problem.

The atlas is the gateway between the brain and the body. No message goes down to the body without passing directly through the atlas and axis. And no message goes up to the brain without passing directly through the same physical opening.

In this way, the upper cervical spine is the power source or communication gateway for your body.

Already, I hope that it is clear that an upper cervical subluxation has the potential to cause a huge number of problems that people do not associate with the neck. In the next chapter we will examine further how spinal tension creates the phenomenon of body imbalance, which may be one of the most common causes of non-traumatic physical injury.

CHAPTER 5

Is Your Head on Straight?

The path of least resistance is what makes
rivers and men crooked.

Dr BJ Palmer

Imagine that you are driving along a highway when a small yellow light starts blinking on your dashboard. Thankfully, you are soon able to find a garage and mechanic.

"No problem," the mechanic says. "Come back in 30 minutes and I'll have the problem fixed for you."

You go away, have a bite to eat, stretch your legs, and return 30 minutes later. You put your keys in the ignition and start the car. Lo-and-behold, the light does not come back on.

"Great!" you exclaim. "What was wrong? How did you fix it?"

"Oh," the mechanic responds, "The problem was that you had a yellow light blinking on your dashboard. I just took the bulb out."

━━━━━━━━━━━━━━━━

Clearly, this mechanic has not done you a favour. Sadly, this is the medical paradigm that so many people follow when it comes to their health: treat the effect but ignore the cause.

The law of cause and effect is one of the most fundamental principles of physics. For every effect in the known universe, there is an original action or cause.

Dr Hannah and Kevin described an extreme array of symptoms that Joe was suffering. Despite receiving the royal treatment at the hospital with CT and MRI testing, no medical doctor or specialist could identify the cause of the problem.

Too many times in my own practice, I have heard stories from people, who have seen countless specialists and have spent thousands of dollars on tests, x-rays, CTs, MRIs and other tests only to be told, "There is nothing wrong with you," or "It's all in your head."

I remember one woman in particular, who had been suffering pain in her entire body for five years. To see me, she had travelled over 1600 kilometres (1000 miles) with a 20 Kg (25 lb) suitcase stuffed with her medical records! She said the same thing: "They can't find anything wrong."

Crazy, isn't it?

━━━━━━━━━━━━━━━━

Let me be abundantly clear: I am not anti-medical. When it comes to things like emergency care, acute illness, disease and surgery, western medicine achieves amazing results and saves lives every day.

However, when it comes to things like headaches, sciatica, fibromyalgia, cancer, hypertension or inflammatory bowel problems, western medicine is often no better than the mechanic, who fixes a problem by removing the blinking bulb

Symptoms are the body's natural way of saying, "There is a problem. Help me!"

While medication reduces symptoms by numbing the body's nerves (e.g., painkillers) or altering the body's biochemistry (e.g., cholesterol lowering medication), they do not correct the cause of the problem.

Healing does not occur from the outside in. It occurs from the inside out. The role of the doctor is to facilitate the healing process by removing the cause of disease in the first place.

Whether the problem is structural, psychological or biochemical in nature, the cause of disease must be addressed for any person to get well.

Upper Cervical chiropractors focus on one specific type of problem that can have multiple effects. Because a subluxation affects the transmission of healing messages from the source (the brainstem), it has the potential to affect the health and function of the entire body.

By correcting the subluxation, Upper Cervical doctors simply facilitate the innate mechanisms of the human body to heal from the inside out.

As spoken by Dr Daniel Kuhn, "When you correct the cause, and you correct the vertebral subluxation, [people] get well." [xxxiv]

In this chapter, we will consider the early signs that a person has a subluxation. Many of these early signs are quite obvious not only to Upper Cervical chiropractors, but even to untrained adults and children.

Interestingly however, the person may not be experiencing any symptoms at all! To see how that is possible, we will consider how spinal tension affects the proprioception pathways.

Proprioception

Let's look again at the location of the tracts within the spinal cord (Figure 5.1).

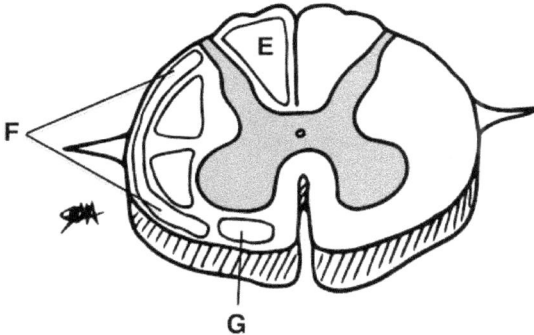

Figure 5.1 More Wires within the Spinal Cord.
E. Dorsal Columns. F. Spinocerebellar Tracts.
G. Reticulospinal Tract.

The dorsal columns (5.1e) and the spinocerebellar tracts (5.1f) are functionally similar. They are the proprioception pathways of the body. Recall from Chapter 1 that proprioception is an unconscious, internal feedback system used to coordinate movement and to maintain balance and posture.

Both the dorsal columns and spinocerebellar tracts transmit signals from the body to the brainstem and the cerebellum. They communicate all messages of spatial positioning, movement and internal body awareness.

The reticulospinal tracts (5.1g) are also proprioception pathways. However, they transmit signals in the opposite direction from brain to the body. They communicate messages of balance and coordination so that your muscles work smoothly.

The proprioception pathways are essential for proper body function.

Recall that less than 0.01% of all neural traffic in the brain enters our conscious awareness. These are the messages related to the motor and sensory pathways. The remaining 99.99% of unconscious processing is related to the proprioception pathways.

The motor and sensory pathways are protected deep inside the cord while the proprioception pathways are unprotected and superficial. Considering this arrangement, there are three important things to consider.

First, an upper cervical problem that affects the spinal cord usually affects the superficial part first: i.e., the proprioception pathways.

Second, because these pathways have such a profound influence on the brain, the problem will likely effect the whole body—not just the neck.

Third, people usually have no idea that there is a problem because the proprioceptive messages are unconscious. It is only after the problem penetrates deeper into the cord does it affect the motor or sensory pathways. It is only then that people become acutely aware that something is wrong.

Body Imbalance

As we've addressed already, an upper cervical subluxation causes a head-neck imbalance (Figure 5.2). Remember also that the brainstem—the command centre that coordinates all messages between the brain and the body—must be level with respect to gravity in order to function properly.

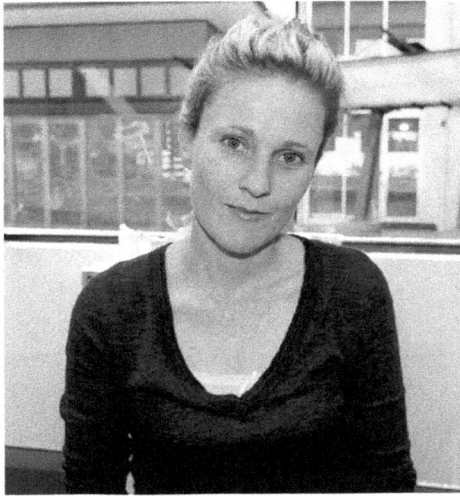

Figure 5.2 Head Tilt.

As noted by Roger Sperry, the 1981 Nobel Prize winner for brain research, "Better than 90% of the brain's output is directed towards maintaining your body in its gravitational field."

If your atlas is unable to support the weight of your head (4.0 – 5.0 Kg), your body will do whatever it takes to find a new balancing point to ensure that your brainstem remains level.

One of the first things that your brain does is call into action the muscles along the front of the neck. Although this action does help to maintain the relative balance of the bowling ball atop your shoulders, it does not come without two significant consequences:

- Straightening of the neck curve or even a reversed-curve (Figure 5.3), and
- Forward head carriage (Figure 5.4).

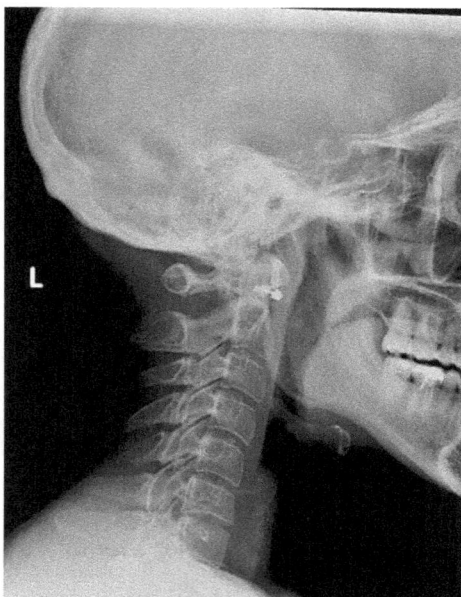

Figure 5.3 Straightening of the Neck Curve on X-Ray.

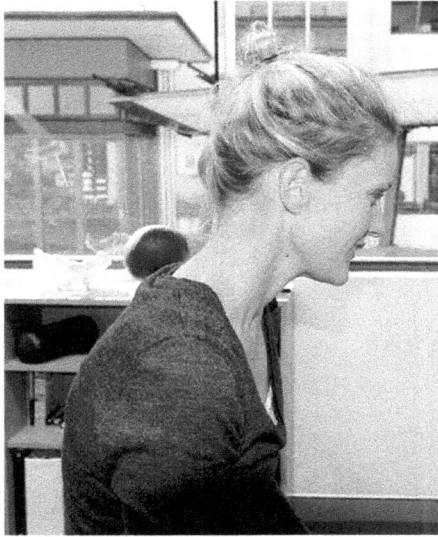

Figure 5.4 Forward Head Carriage.

On an x-ray, the normal curve of the neck is described as lordotic or forward facing with an arc of 31-40 degrees. xxxv This curve correlates with the tilt of the atlas as it maintains the balance of the head.

As your neck straightens and your head extends forward beyond the tip of your shoulder, it creates major stress across the muscles and ligaments that connect your head to your back. In fact, for every 2.5 cm of forward head carriage, the weight of your head doubles. xxxvi

So if your head is jutting forward by 2.5 cm (one inch), the effective weight of your head becomes 10 Kg (21 pounds). If your head is really protruding forward by 5.0 cm, the effective weight increases to 20 Kg (42 pounds)!

Forward head carriage is one of the most significant causes of illness and injury. It is also one of the major reasons that people experience chronic muscle soreness in their neck, back and shoulders.

A straightened neck curve also exerts great pressure on your spinal cord. If this tension affects the proprioception pathways (which is quite likely), it creates muscle tightness, postural abnormalities and a phenomenon known as body imbalance (Figure 5.5).

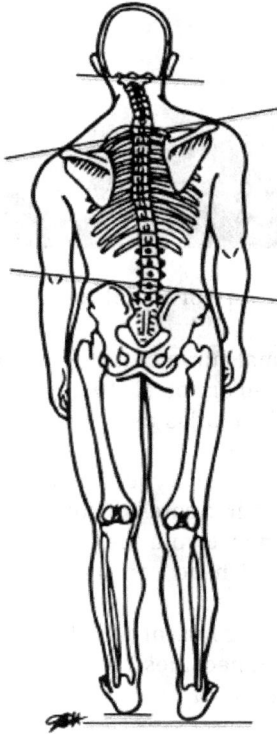

Figure 5.5 Body Imbalance.

Body imbalance is the automatic process by which your body adapts in order to minimize spinal tension but also to maintain head equilibrium.

Because body imbalance is an automatic process, you may never realise the problem until someone else comments on it or until you look in a mirror.

You may notice that your head protrudes forward or tilts to one side.

You may remark that your shoulders roll forward and appear uneven.

You may feel lopsided when you walk or notice that one of your feet slaps the ground harder than the other one.

You may see that your hips are twisted, which causes one of your legs to be drawn upward. You may even have an abnormal spinal curvature. xxxvii xxxviii xxxix

If you are lying on a table or bed, it may appear that one of your legs is shorter than the other. This sign of body imbalance commonly called a leg length inequality (LLI) or short leg is one of the most accurate indicators used by Upper Cervical chiropractors to determine if you have an atlas subluxation. This assessment will be described in greater detail in Chapter 17.

In short, you will see that your body is crooked even though it feels like you are straight!

———————

Case Report: Running Injuries

My wife, Natalie and I both have a passion for trail running.

As amateur athletes, we regularly pay attention to our bodies' signs and symptoms to make sure that we are not doing something that may lead to an injury.

One year before Natalie and I met, she had suffered an episode of plantar fasciitis. Plantar fasciitis (PF) is caused by inflammation of the tendons on the sole of the foot. The burning pain that Natalie felt along her left arch forced her onto the sidelines for a couple of months (which feels like an eternity for a runner). Eventually the problem did resolve on its own, but Natalie would still experience the odd twinge now and again.

It was unfortunate that only a few weeks after we started dating, she suffered a major relapse. This time, however, it was in her right foot. Additionally, she was experiencing a stabbing pain along the outside of her left knee and leg.

At first, we thought this new problem was tightness of her iliotibial band (ITB), which is the tendon that connects the hip/buttock muscles to the outside of the knee. After a more thorough assessment, however, we realised that the problem was actually a mild sprain of her tibio-fibular ligament between her leg and ankle.

The strange thing about the situation was that Natalie stretched quite religiously. Neither her ITB nor her PF nor any other muscle or ligament was tight at all. On the other hand, her ankle joint was exceptionally rigid.

The ankle joints are like the body's shock absorbers. If the joints are jammed, they cannot absorb shock. As a consequence, the extra force that comes with every footfall can cause a number of problems: shin splints, calf strains, Achilles sprains and an extensive array of knee injuries.

I offered to adjust Natalie, who had never tried chiropractic. Although her neck was tight and although she did have a considerable leg length inequality, I thought they were the secondary effects of the lower limb problem.

I was still relatively new in chiropractic practice, and because Natalie was a runner, I assumed that the cause of her injuries must have been somewhere in the lower half of her body.

Alas, one month later and despite my best efforts, Natalie was not doing much better. Therefore, we decided to try what we should have done first: an atlas adjustment.

Within one week of Natalie's first adjustment, we noticed dramatic improvements. For the past month, Natalie could not run further than 5 km without succumbing to unbearable foot and knee pain.

That first week, Natalie was able to run without any pain, and she doubled her distance to 10 km. A couple of weeks later, she was comfortably running a half-marathon (21 km) again.

Overuse and repetitive stress may certainly have contributed toward Natalie's injuries.

However, it is quite remarkable that it was not until her upper neck was adjusted that she was able to recover.

Had I been better versed in the concept of body imbalance at the time, I may not have waited so long to try an Upper Cervical treatment for an injury so far away from the neck.

Time and experience are great teachers!

As I would research later, body imbalance that creates a leg length inequality of 1.5 cm may be sufficient to trigger problems in a non-athlete. However, because the force of each footfall is greater with athletes, an imbalance as small as 0.5 cm may be sufficient to spark injury. [xl]

No matter how large or small the imbalance, asymmetrical stress that persists long enough will result in injury. It is really only a matter of time and repetition until it happens.

Natalie and I continue to be checked and adjusted regularly. Although we run marathons, seldom do we need to take any time off due to injury. It makes you wonder how well athletes of any calibre — professional, amateur, casual or even beginner—may do with proper Upper Cervical care.

CHAPTER 6

Your Body is Crooked

What you are speaks so loud that
I cannot hear what you say.

Ralph Waldo Emerson

Imagine that you find yourself in some B-rated movie. You have been kidnapped by a madman, who has strapped a bomb to your chest. The mad bomber takes you to the middle of some field and then hands you two small objects.

In your left hand is an object the size of a large water bottle (750 mL). In your right hand is an object the size of a small water bottle (400 mL).

The mad bomber explains that these objects are detonators. He warns you that you must keep these detonators elevated 1 metre above the ground or else the bombs will explode. He also warns that the bombs will explode if you let go of them for even a second.

Despite your dire situation, the madman offers you a glimmer of hope. He informs you that there is a town 80 km (50 miles) straight west, and in the town is a police station. He also informs you that any bomb technician should be able to disarm the chest rig. All you have to do is survive long enough to get help.

The mad bomber cackles with sinister delight and then leaves you on your own.

(Yes, this scenario is completely absurd, and why he is doing it I have no idea. Just play along anyway. I promise that there is a point to it all.)

In the first few minutes, you cry desperately for help. As your rational mind returns, you realise that your only chance to survive is to start walking. You know it will be hard, but you do believe it is within your power to make it. All you will have to do is hold onto the detonators and make sure that they stay elevated 1 metre above the ground.

Within the first hour of walking (or maybe running), you begin to feel the asymmetrical stress as the detonators weigh heavily on your arms. For as light as the two detonators are, you really start to feel their weight.

You shift your position to rest your hands on the back of your neck. Shortly thereafter, you begin to feel the strain on your shoulders, so you change back to holding the detonators outward at your sides.

As much as you wish you could switch hands exchange the weights for a bit of balance, you know that you cannot release them or else the bomb will explode.

After a few hours of walking, the tension through your arms and shoulders has descended all the way through your back and legs. Despite the burning pain and heaviness of your muscles, you march onward knowing that you must survive.

I think you get the idea by now.

Stepping back into reality, there are a few important things that this absurd situation illustrates as it relates to body imbalance.

The bomb and the detonators represent your head and your brain. Your body will do whatever it takes to keep them upright, even if it means sacrificing itself to do so.

The asymmetrical weight represents the stress caused by an upper neck misalignment. If there is an imbalance, your body will experience far greater stress than if the weights were balanced.

Finally, the bomb technician (whom we never met in our story) represents an Upper Cervical chiropractor. A subluxation is often a relatively simple problem to correct with the proper knowhow. However, it still requires that you seek help before he or she can do anything about it.

Body imbalance is an interesting, phenomenon to observe. However, the consequences of chronic imbalance may be quite serious.

A common thing that people say when they come to my office the first time is, "I didn't do anything to cause my problem." These people usually add that they were doing something innocent like stepping off a ladder, turning their head while driving, or sitting at a desk. Then suddenly they were unable to turn their necks, move their arms or even stand upright without experiencing intense pain.

Although your atlas may be subluxated, you may not notice the problem for weeks, months or even years after the problem first appeared.

It is like the straw that breaks the camel's back. Or it is like continuously stretching an elastic band: if you do it often enough, there will come a time when it loses its elasticity and snaps.

Similarly, if you have the chronic, cumulative stress of body imbalance for a long enough time, all it may take is one innocent thing that finally causes something in your body to break.

Chronic stress causes muscles to ache, burn and eventually tear.

Chronic stress causes ligaments to stretch, swell and snap.

Chronic stress causes joints to rust, erode and break.

And chronic stress causes organs to fatigue, fail and eventually die.

In this way, an atlas subluxation may cause you to suffer arthritis, bursitis, tendonitis, sprains or strains, [xli] [xlii] frozen joints, [xliii] [xliv] cartilage damage, [xlv] spinal disc damage, [xlvi] [xlvii] [xlviii] [xlix] muscles soreness, heaviness, restlessness, chronic fatigue symptoms or fibromyalgia. [l] [li] [lii] [liii]

Case Report: Intercostal Neuralgia

Mark was an active farmer in his late 60s, who had to drive over 5-hours to visit my office. He had no great expectations but figured it was worth a shot to see if I could help him.

Mark proceeded to describe an intense shooting pain through the middle of his back at the level of the 10th thoracic vertebra, which radiated along his ribs and into his chest. The problem was greatly affecting everything in his daily life from driving his tractor (especially in reverse) to walking down a hill.

I asked Mark if he had ever noticed a rash, which may have suggested that he had been suffering an ongoing case of shingles

"Never," he answered. "This has been going on for almost a year, and its getting worse. I've been referred for x-rays, ultrasounds of my liver and pancreas and CAT scans, but they can't find anything except a bit of arthritis. My doc says he thinks there's something else besides the arthritis that's causing it, but he doesn't know what it could be. I've been to all the physios and chiros within 50 kilometres. And I've been to all the specialists in the city, but none of them have been able to help me.

"The reason I've come to see you is because you were able to help my niece. I'm hoping you've got one more miracle for an old man like me."

"Miracles?" I laughed in response. "Probably not, but I'll do the best I can."

Mark's problem sounded like intercostal neuralgia, which is caused when the spinal nerve roots between the ribs are inflamed. It is like waving your hand over an open fire. Any twisting or sudden movement that aggravates the inflamed area irritates the nerve and triggers the pain.

The thing about intercostal neuralgia is that it is not an uncommon problem. It responds very well with a number of therapies including massage, physiotherapy and chiropractic. I would have expected at least one of Mark's health providers to have been able to treat the problem.

Then again, that would only be true if Mark's problem was a simple case of intercostal neuralgia.

Mark's neck was quite rigid around the atlas. Aside from insomnia and the odd headache,

Mark denied ever having any issues with his neck.

I was not surprised. As Dr Tom Forest explains, "One-third of the nerves [in the upper neck] produce pain when they're pinched. Two-thirds of them don't.

"So you see, two-thirds of the people are walking around like this," he says, tilting his head to one side and shrugging his shoulder upward, "saying, 'I don't need a chiropractor. I feel fine.' And they feel fine because the body has produced certain chemicals to deaden the nerves. Otherwise we would all just have unrelenting pain." [liv]

As I checked Mark for signs of body imbalance, I discovered the likely source of his problem: his left leg appeared to be 3 cm shorter than his right. I took a picture to show Mark, who was flabbergasted. Aside from his rib pain, Mark had never experienced any injuries or any troubles with his legs or lower back at all.

In fact, the only injury that he could recall was a severe car accident when he was in his 20s where he smashed his head through a windscreen. "There wasn't any blood, but I still went to the hospital anyway. They didn't think I broke anything, so they just sent me home. It's just how it was done those days."

I say it often that just because there aren't any broken bones, or just because there isn't any blood, that doesn't mean that everything is okay.

I explained the phenomenon of body imbalance, and also how something that happened a long time ago can still cause problems years down the track.

"The spine is like a chain link," I explained. "If you twist the first link, it can cause a chain reaction, which affects all the other ones. With enough stress and time, though, those links start to break down.

"If your spine was made of metal, we'd call it 'rust.' But because your spine is made of bone, we call it 'arthritis.'

"It isn't the vertebra causing all the trouble that usually gets the arthritis. It is the one bearing the extra stress. So your T10 vertebra is most likely just the weak link in the chain.

"It is your atlas and probably your car accident that actually started this problem all those years ago. That's why no one else can figure it out."

I could see the light bulb turn on inside Mark's head. He insisted that we get started with treatment right away. After taking an x-ray to see what was going on, I was able to adjust him. Although there was little palpable difference with his neck, his leg length inequality dropped to just a couple of millimetres. Not a bad change for 2 minutes worth of work!

Mark was visiting family for the next week, so I advised he should return for a checkup in a couple of days.

He returned 24 hours later. I was not sure what to make of his unexpected arrival until I realised that he was attempting to withhold a smile from me.

Mark started. "Last night was the first night's sleep I've had in months that my back hasn't woken me up." He added that his neck felt almost exactly the same; but aside from a bit of muscle soreness, his middle back and ribs were almost completely pain free.

A regular 10-hour round trip to my office was never a viable option, so after checking him a couple more times that week, I instructed him to call me if ever he felt a flare up. It was two weeks before I heard from Mark, and the next time was over a month.

I usually see Mark once every 3 months for a checkup, and he is still as active as ever. Although it is not practical for him to pursue the full amount of treatment he requires to truly fix his problem, the fact that his condition has stabilised so well with such minimal intervention is a wonderful reminder that it is always better to do something than nothing at all.

Moreover, Mark's case is an important reminder that there is not always a connection between the location of your symptoms and the location of the actual problem.

Symptoms can be misleading.

> As Dr Forest reminds us, "Upper Cervical is based upon the premise that when the atlas dislodges and it can't pull itself back in, it can create the vast array of problems. And rather than focusing on adjusting where the pain is located, we focus on getting back to where the epicentre is." [lv]

━━━━━━━━━━━━━━━━━━━━━━━

Dr Daniel Clark, an Upper Cervical doctor and educator, summarizes the process of body imbalance very well. "When the weight of the head is moved off the centre at the top of the neck because of head tilt, the rest of the body will begin to compensate for that shift of weight. One shoulder will come down, a hip is brought up, bringing a leg up with it creating body imbalance." [lvi]

Body imbalance caused by an upper cervical subluxation creates spinal tension, physical stress and potential damage to all tissues in the body.

Body imbalance is one of the earliest signs of an upper cervical problem. Most importantly, it usually appears long before a person ever senses or feels that there is a problem.

I often hear people say, "I don't have any pain. There's nothing wrong with me." The problem is that they say so with a crooked head.

To modify the quotation at the beginning of this chapter, your body speaks so loud that I cannot hear what you say.

As a final thought for this chapter, you may want to look in the mirror yourself. Is your head on straight?

CHAPTER 7

The Power Source

All the drugs in the world cannot adjust a subluxated vertebra.

Dr BJ Palmer

———————

I don't know who I expected Joe to be. Maybe a middle aged or elderly man. Maybe someone who was a bit overweight or looking very sickly.

Whatever I was expecting, I certainly did not expect to see Joe for who he was: a healthy-looking young man in his mid 20s.

Someone just like me ... except that the person lying in front of me was clenched into a fetal position, shivering, clenching his eyes shut firmly, and grimacing in agony.

That little voice inside my head started to panic again.

How are x-rays going to help if he's already had MRIs and other tests at the hospital? What if they missed something? What if Dad is wrong?

"Any changes, Joe?" Dr Hannah asked as he stepped into the room.

"I haven't felt nauseous for a while," Joe replied softly pointing to a bucket nearest the head of the table. "The room is still spinning, but as long as I keep my eyes closed I can tolerate it."

"Joe, this is my son, Jeffrey."

"Hi," was the only word that I could weakly articulate.

Fortunately, my dad was able to continue for me. "Jeffrey works in the radiology department. I've asked him to see if we can get you in for those x-rays we talked about."

"Thank you."

How helpless and desperate Joe must have been feeling that morning I will never know. The exhaustion yet earnest appreciation was apparent in his voice.

The entire time at Palmer, I had been a timid student doing only what my superiors told me. My classmates and I had been taught that chiropractic was only good for the relief of neck, lower back and similar musculoskeletal pain.

We had also been warned that if we ever treated anyone with any other condition that we would be going beyond the scope of our practice and could lose our licenses.

To be honest, I did not think that an x-ray would make any difference. I did not believe that Upper Cervical would do anything at all to help.

What could an Upper Cervical adjustment possibly do to help this poor guy?

I asked myself this question many times that morning.

I felt utterly powerless. However, I knew also that to deny Joe any hope would have been the most terrible thing I could have done. I felt compelled to do something.

It was as if the universe had brought me into this moment to give me a choice: to act in spite of my personal doubts and fears—to become a real doctor—or to remain as I had always been and to do nothing.

In hindsight, I think I chose well.

"Okay," I said to Joe and my dad, "I'll do down to radiology and see what I can do."

———————

I am a far different chiropractor today than I was back then. Still I would be a fool to believe that I have seen and done it all. There are many Upper Cervical doctors in the world far more skilled and knowledgeable than I.

I have much yet to learn.

I agree with a quote that is attributed to Socrates, "I am the wisest man alive, for I know one thing, and that is that I know nothing."

The energy fields and innate mechanisms by which the body sustains itself are far beyond my understanding and expertise. Fortunately, I understand just enough that I know how to work with these forces in order to help people heal. I also have just enough experience that my old doubts and fears of working with incurable or impossible cases have been replaced with faith and hope.

By now it should be clear that an atlas problem has the potential to cause problems anywhere in the body. In this final chapter on neuroanatomy, we will examine how an upper cervical problem affects the brainstem, which impacts not only your muscles and joints, but your organs as well and even your mind.

———————

The Command Centre

The brainstem is the command centre for your nervous system (Figure 7.1). Like the spinal cord, it is divided into neuron clusters and wires. Unlike the cord, the boundaries and functions of these neurons and tracts are infinitely more complex.

If your spinal cord is like an airport in the middle of the desert, your brainstem is like the air-traffic control room for NASA. Fortunately, a surface examination of the brainstem will be more than sufficient for our purposes.

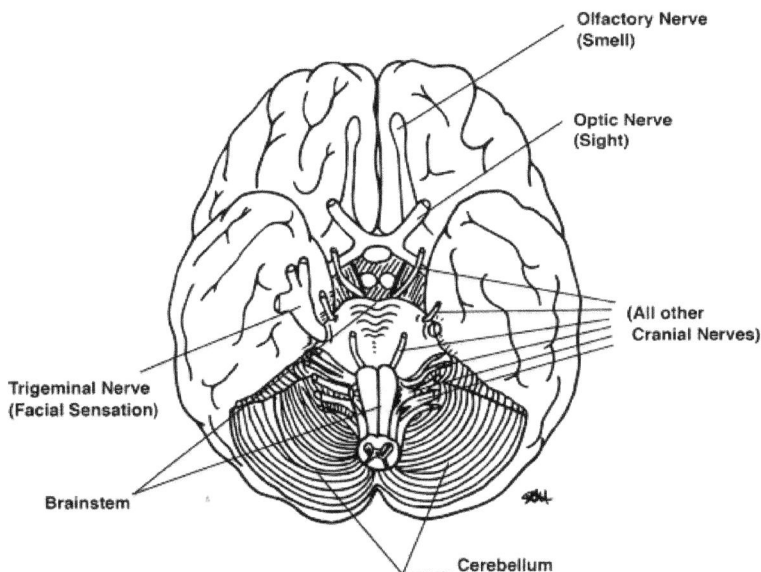

Figure 7.1 Undersurface of the Brain and Brainstem.

The brainstem is the origin site for ten of the 12 pairs of cranial nerves. These nerves control movement and receive sensory information from the head and face. The cranial nerves also receive the special sensory information of smell, sight, hearing, balance and taste.

The brainstem also includes a large cluster of neurons that transmit messages for all the autonomic or automatic processes that happen inside your body:

- the rhythmic beating of your heart;
- the circulation of blood throughout your tissues;
- the movement of air into and out of your lungs;
- the digestion of food and the absorption of nutrients;

- the elimination of waste products;
- the maintenance of your blood pressure; and
- the function of your immune system, to name just a few.

Not only do these autonomic neurons regulate organ functions, they also regulate the biochemistry of your blood. In other words, they monitor and maintain the proper level of oxygen, vitamins, minerals, hormones and neurotransmitters that allow your body to work.

Case Report: Bell's Palsy

One of the most remarkable transformations I have ever seen with Upper Cervical care was the case of a woman named Anne, who was one of my dad's patients at Palmer.

I have never met Anne in person. Instead, this case report is about a video that my younger sister (who is also a chiropractor) recorded with Anne's permission.

Anne was involved in a horrific motor vehicle accident that left her with serious neurological complications including left-sided facial paralysis. Her medical doctors, neurologists and spinal surgeons wrote-off her condition as Bell's palsy, which they believed was caused by permanent nerve damage.

What troubled Anne was that she knew that she had not suffered permanent nerve damage. Her reasoning was simple: when she rotated her head to the extreme left, her facial paralysis completely disappeared!

When she sought my dad's expertise for another opinion, he recommended that she should have an Upper Cervical x-ray. For all his years in practise, even he was surprised with what he saw. The normal total rotational movement between the atlas and the skull bone is 5 degrees.

Anne's atlas had misaligned, in fact dislocated by over 40 degrees!

The video that my sister recorded is only about 60 seconds long, but it is shocking, if not a little frightening to watch.

It starts with Anne before an Upper Cervical treatment. Her voice is soft and gravelly. She has complete left-sided facial drooping, and she is unable to smile evenly, move or even open her left eye.

Anne then lies on her side for the treatment, and then sits upright again.

Nothing happens for about five seconds until you see a quiver and then a twitch in Anne's cheek and upper lip. Next, her eyelids flicker, and she blinks rapidly. Finally with a deep yawn followed by a sigh, you see a different woman appear. Her voice is full and clear. She has even muscle tone on both sides of her face, and she is able to smile and move her eyes normally.

All these changes happened within a span of 10 seconds. When Dr Hannah first adjusted Anne, this transformation would last only a few minutes. Over time as Anne's body healed, however, the adjustment would hold for a few days at a time.

Given the severity of Anne's injury, it is unlikely that she will ever recover completely from her injuries. It is likely that she will require regular Upper Cervical care for the rest of her life.

However, the video of her physical transformation should be a strong reminder for patients, doctors and specialists everywhere that no disease or condition should ever be regarded as incurable or impossible.

The power that made the body heals the body. All it needs it the chance to do so.

―――――――――――――――

The lifeblood to the brainstem flows through a pair of arteries known as the vertebral arteries (Figure 7.2).

These arteries run through the sides of the 6th cervical vertebra (C6) all the way to the head. Up to the level of the axis, the vertebral arteries follow a relatively straight route. Thereafter, the arteries make a series of twists. After looping forward from C2 through C1, the arteries twirl backward around the ring of the atlas and then back onto the front of the brainstem where they unite to form the basilar artery.

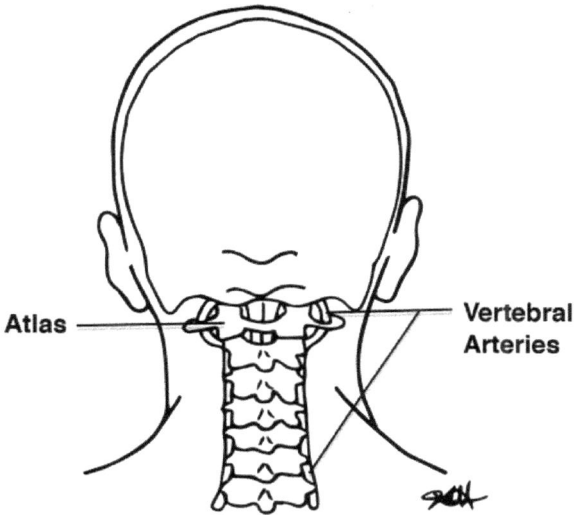

Figure 7.2 The Vertebral Arteries.

Like a garden hose, the arteries are strong and flexible. Unless they are damaged in some way, they do not tear even when they are under high amounts of stress, most notably when you rotate and fully extend your head.

Combined, these blood vessels supply 30% of the total blood to the brain. However, they supply 99% of the blood to the brainstem and the cerebellum. [lvii]

As you may recall, between the cerebellum (60 billion) and the brainstem (20 billion), these two critical structures account for 80% of all neurons in the human brain. To reiterate as well, these neurons control all the primal, unconscious functions of life.

The take-home message is that the vertebral arteries provide the life-blood for 80% of all the nerve cells in your brain.

CHAPTER 8

Cutting the Power

*When health is absent wisdom cannot reveal itself,
art cannot become manifest, strength cannot be ex-
erted, wealth is useless and reason is powerless.*

Herophiles

Think of the garden hose again with water flowing out of a noz-
zle. If you were to create a kink in the hose, step on it or exert
tension on it in any other way, it should be no surprise that the
flow of water would stop.

Like your foot on a hose, a subluxation may disrupt the flow of
blood to the brainstem (Figure 8.1). Usually it is not so much that
the whole brain suffocates, but just enough that you will certainly
suffer consequences.

When we consider the cranial nerves and the autonomic neurons of the brainstem, it should be no surprise that there is a vast array of problems that may occur.

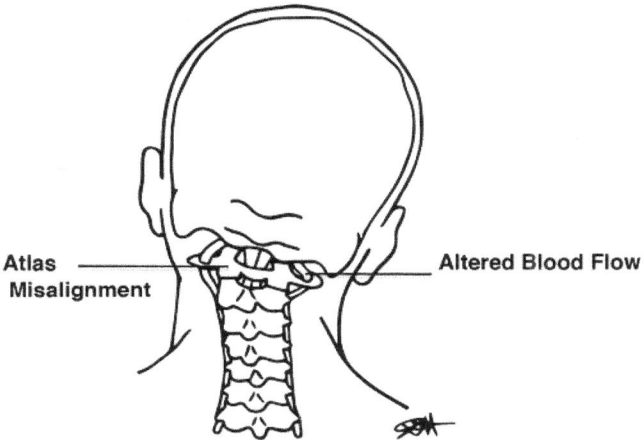

Figure 8.1 Altered Blood Flow Through the Vertebral Arteries

The 1st cranial nerve controls the sense of smell, and the 2nd cranial nerve receives all messages from the eyes that relate to light, motion, and colour. The 3rd, 4th and 6th cranial nerves work together to control the small muscles that move the eyes.

The 1st and 2nd cranial nerves do not originate from the brainstem itself, but from the cerebral cortex (upper portion of the brain). However, both nerves communicate with other neurons located within the brainstem. Thus, a circulatory problem that affects these neurons may affect the senses of smell and sight.

When an upper neck problem affects the flow of blood to the brainstem, you may suffer visual disturbances such as double vision, blurriness, crossed-eyes or other problems that affect your ability to focus or move your eyes. [lviii lix lx lxi lxii]

The 7th cranial nerve receives all messages of taste. These nerves also control all muscles of facial expression with the exception of the jaw muscles. Those muscles are controlled by the 5th cranial nerves, which also receive all the sensory information about temperature, pressure and pain from the face.

Skipping ahead, the 11th cranial nerve controls the sternocleido-mastoid and trapezius, two major muscles that move the head neck and shoulders. The 12th cranial nerve controls all muscles that move the tongue.

Accordingly, you may suffer motor contractions, eye twitching, torticollis (aka wry neck) or neck spasms; [lxiii lxiv lxv lxvi] jaw problems (collectively known as temporomandibular disorders or TMD) [lxvii lxviii] or even facial paralysis, which is known as Bell's palsy. [lxix]

The 8th cranial nerve receives all sensory information from the inner ear for balance and hearing.

An atlas problem may cause you to suffer hearing problems, [lxx lxxi lxxii] ear blockages, [lxxiii lxxiv] or even inner ear problems including tinnitus, vertigo or Ménière's disease. [lxxv lxxvi lxxvii lxxviii]

Finally, the 9th and 10th cranial nerves work together to coordinate all muscles in the throat involved with swallowing and speech.

The 10th cranial nerve (also known as the vagus nerve) connects with the autonomic neurons in the brainstem to transmit messages to and from all the organs in your body: the thyroid gland, voice box, lungs, heart, stomach, small and large intestines, liver, gallbladder, pancreas, spleen, kidneys, bladder and reproductive organs.

The nerve also controls a tiny sensor in the neck known as the carotid body, which monitors blood pressure and biochemical levels. In this way, the nerve influences blood flow to the head, brain and the rest of the body.

An upper cervical problem affecting these nerves may contribute toward physiological or organ diseases including abnormal blood pressure (high or low), [lxxix lxxx lxxxi lxxxii lxxxiii lxxxiv] heart and circulatory problems, [lxxxv lxxxvi lxxxvii] fainting spells, [lxxxviii] swallowing or speech problems, breathing problems including asthma, [lxxxix xc xci xcii] bowel problems, [xciii] or other immunological disorders. [xciv xcv xcvi]

I'm sure it is clear that if an upper neck problem affects the cranial nerves, the consequences may be far-reaching. As a final point, consider how your ability to think would be affected if your brain received any less than 100% of its proper blood supply.

Imagine that you place a wet cloth over your mouth. Now try to breathe. It may still be possible, but it is probably much harder to get the same amount of air into your lungs.

It is the same when your brain is starved of oxygen-rich blood. It may continue to function, but its ability to work efficiently and clearly may drop significantly.

As a result, you may suffer neurological symptoms such as light-headedness, "fogginess in the head" or an inability to focus, [xcvii xcviii xcix c] sleeping problems such as insomnia or sleep apnea, epilepsy or similar disorders, [ci cii ciii civ] or other neurological problems such as Parkinson's disease [cv] or multiple sclerosis. [cvi cvii cviii]

You may even suffer attention deficit or hyperactivity disorders (ADD/ADHD) [cix cx cxi] or other behavioural disorders. [cxii cxiii cxiv cxv]

I see it with many of my patients, and I know it myself: when my atlas is misaligned, I do not feel like myself. I become irritable and restless. I don't sleep well. I have a hard time concentrating. In short, I just feel uncomfortable, and I struggle through my day until I get the problem corrected.

Case Report: Epilepsy

Andrew was a man in his 70s with a long history of lower neck problems. Although he was hesitant to see a chiropractor, he decided to give it a shot when the stiffness and pain started to affect his weekly round of golf.

Considering Andrew's age and the fact that he had very significant forward head carriage, I advised that we take an x-ray of his neck. As I expected to see, Andrew had a significant amount of degenerative arthritis and a definite atlas misalignment.

I adjusted Andrew and advised him to come back in a couple of days after he would have an opportunity to go golfing.

When he returned, Andrew described that it was a little easier looking side-to-side, but he added something quite unexpected.

"I don't know what you did, but I think you cured my epilepsy."

"Excuse me?" I asked. I was most surprised because Andrew had failed to report any medical conditions even when I had asked him on his previous visit.

"I didn't tell you, but since I was just a boy I've been diagnosed with epilepsy. Not the seizure kind, but usually around 10 times a day I'll get a 'turn' where I blank out."

Andrew was describing what is known as a petite-mal seizure that occurs if the nervous system is bombarded with too many messages that don't make any sense. Think of it as a time-out mechanism that the brain uses to protect itself.

"I've seen heaps of specialists, had all these tests and been taking epilepsy medication all my life, but none of it has really made any difference. Anyway, that night after you did that thing to my neck, I only had one turn. And the next day I didn't have any!

"I've only had three turns since you did that. I don't know what it is or what you did, but that's made one big difference!"

Over the next several months, Andrew continued with Upper Cervical care, which he reported did two important things. First, it reduced his episodes to less than 10 per week (previously 10 per day). But second, (and possibly more important for Andrew), it allowed him to play not just one, but two rounds of golf per week! pain-free.

Upper cervical neuroanatomy is an immeasurably deep subject, and we have only scratched its surface. For now, these chapters should be more than sufficient to demonstrate how a misalignment of the upper cervical spine can have a profound impact on your health.

Before we completely lose the forest through the trees, I would like to reiterate the simple concepts presented at the very beginning of this book.

The brain controls all messages to every cell in the entire body, including messages of health and healing.

The upper cervical spine—the atlas and the axis—directly affects the spinal cord and the brainstem, which is the control centre of the brain.

If there is a misalignment of the upper cervical spine, the brain is not able to communicate properly with the rest of the body. As a direct consequence, health problems will begin to appear.

Upper Cervical is a specialist approach to chiropractic that corrects the misalignment of the atlas and axis, thereby restoring the health and optimal wellbeing of the body.

If these four sentences are the only things that you have learnt from this book thus far, then I have achieved my goal.

In the next sections, I will discuss how an Upper Cervical problem happens in the first place. I will also explain how an Upper Cervical chiropractor works to correct the problem.

If the first few chapters have seemed a bit overwhelming, rest assured that the remainder of this book is not nearly as technical.

You do not need to be an expert in neuroanatomy to understand Upper Cervical care. However, I do hope that by covering these basics that you may have a stronger appreciation of the science behind it.

Why do I feel it is important?

Because it was the one thing that I did not really understand when I met Joe.

I knew the basics of neuroanatomy and chiropractic; I didn't understand the big picture. Even though I was supposed to be helping Joe, I harboured so many doubts and fears that I did not really know what to do.

How are x-rays going to help if he's already had MRIs and other tests at the hospital? What if they missed something? What if Dad is wrong?

What could Upper Cervical possibly do to help this poor guy?

For as many times as I asked these and other questions, I was about to see for myself.

Part II

Philosophy

Interlude I

What is called genius is the abundance of life and health.

Henry David Thoreau

————————

I've been under chiropractic care for as long as I can remember. However, you may find it interesting to learn that until I was 25 years old, the style of chiropractic that I preferred was general spinal manipulation.

Throughout my younger life, I had three recurring problems that required regular treatment: my left shoulder that I had injured numerous times playing football, wrestling and lifting weights when I was in my teens; my right pelvic (sacroiliac or SI) joint that would flare up for no good reason when I started running in my early 20s; and my upper neck (C2) that was likely related to studying too much through high school and university.

Having a parent who is a chiropractor definitely has its perks! Whether I was suffering a headache, sports injury, or if I was just feeling off, my dad was always there to "fix me."

As far as spinal manipulation went, the cracking never bothered me, and I would always feel fantastic after an adjustment. As a patient, I always knew that chiropractic works. For many years that was all I needed to know.

However, there was one significant problem: my adjustments would never hold in place. Holding is a term used by chiropractors to describe the length of time that a vertebra stays in its normal alignment.

Alas, three times per week I would need my dad to put my body back together.

To complicate the situation, I was a chiropractic student. Spinal instability or hypermobility is a common problem for many young chiropractors, who learn spinal manipulation by practicing on each other. It often takes several years before many chiropractors recover from the physical abuse that they suffer as a part of their education.

I was fortunate that one of my first contacts when I moved to Australia was Dr Joe Ierano, an Upper Cervical chiropractor who remains one of my closest mentors today. One of the many ways that Joe helped me in my early days was by introducing Dr Bryce Conrad, who was looking to hire an associate chiropractor at the time.

For two years with Bryce's guidance and support, I practiced a combination of Upper Cervical and general chiropractic. Although my career was only beginning, I knew already that my focus would be shifting away from the style of chiropractic that I had always known and more toward Upper Cervical care.

Under Bryce and Joe's care, I also became an Upper Cervical patient myself. Although I still suffered my regular niggles, I was noticing a remarkable change that by receiving fewer manual treatments, my adjustments were holding longer. I found myself going a week without needing an adjustment.

Something was definitely working!

A twisted series of events would transpire over the next several months, which would find me in a different state and starting my own practice. With Bryce and Joe 1000km away (and my dad over 10,000km away), I found myself for the first time in my life without a chiropractor.

Again, I was fortunate that another of my Upper Cervical mentors, Dr Darren Scheuner, practiced only 100km away. Alas, the challenge would be and remains finding the time to visit him!

I came to rely heavily on my wife Natalie, who was studying massage therapy at the time. She was also able to help me to adjust my own atlas using an Upper Cervical instrument. For nearly 6-months, this bastardized but effective version of Upper Cervical care was the only type of treatment that I received.

The amazing thing was that I was doing better than ever.

First, two weeks passed without any problems. Then a whole month passed. Then another month. All the while I kept asking myself, "Why isn't my back hurting?" In the past, I could only run 20 kilometres before my right SI joint started to throb. Now I was running marathons without any injuries at all.

For me, Upper Cervical care has allowed my body to do the one thing that it was never able to do in all the years I had with general spinal manipulation: heal.

I believe that a number of other factors have contributed to my increased stability and wellbeing including better dietary habits, regular exercise and regular massage for those minor muscle aches.

Nevertheless, having seen the same thing with my own patients that they are feeling great and that their treatments are holding longer than ever, I am convinced that it is Upper Cervical care that has made the most profound difference.

The Three Enemies of Progress

After reading the stories and science in the first part of this book, you may be wondering why you have never heard any of it before. If Upper Cervical care is so amazing, why isn't it on the cover on every magazine, on every health blog and on every television show that you see?

You may also be wondering why your doctor has never mentioned Upper Cervical care to you.

According to Dr Robert Brooks, the answer is three-fold. "Ignorance, which is just not knowing. Prejudice, which is believing something that isn't true. And superstition, which is something that would keep you from investigating something that might really help you." [cxvi]

Ignorance (simply not knowing) is a problem that affects both the public and other health practitioners including medical doctors, specialists and allied health therapists. The problem even extends to other chiropractors, who may have never heard about Upper Cervical care.

It is mind-boggling that Upper Cervical care is scarcely mentioned at any chiropractic university in Australia.

As a former supervisor with Macquarie University in Sydney, I will testify to this bewildering omission. I recall many conversations with students and other supervisors, who ask about my practice.

Every time I would give the same answer: "Upper Cervical."

And every time I would receive the same blank stare and response: "Upper Cervical? What's that?"

No matter how many times I heard it, it never ceased to amaze me!

I believe that the overall problem of ignorance is best summarized by one Upper Cervical patient, who is quoted as saying, "I have seen at least 20 chiropractors, 10 surgeons, 18 medical doctors, 15 physical therapists, 4 acupuncturists, 18 massage therapists and spent thousands of dollars over 38 years ... No one has ever suggested I try Upper Cervical care!" [cxvii]

Prejudice is the second problem. It is unfortunate that the propaganda and opinions of cynics and nay-sayers are so loud that many people never get to hear the truth from the Upper Cervical researchers and experts who achieve real results every day.

Chiropractic prejudice often follows one of three arguments: that it is unregulated, that is it unsafe or that it is unscientific. These three points will be addressed throughout this book. Certainly, there are documented cases of people who have had strong negative experiences with chiropractic. The same can be said for all professions from solicitors and medical doctors to bookkeepers and electricians.

Some people are simply more skilled than others. However, when you consider the exceptional track record of Upper Cervical care and the large body of evidence to support it—not only the hundreds of clinical trials, studies and case reports, but also the thousands of life changing testimonials—it should be become quickly clear that any prejudices against Upper Cervical care are quite unfound.

———————————

Superstition is a problem where I am just as guilty as the next person. As you have likely gathered from reading my account of Joe's story, I did not believe that an Upper Cervical treatment would help him at all.

Although I had studied Upper Cervical theory and heard a handful of wonderful stories, I had never seen any of it with my own eyes. I believed that there was no way that one atlas misalignment could cause so many extreme problems.

In all honesty, I believed that those stories were just coincidences, superstitions and myths.

Many things have changed in my life since that time. I can now testify not only as a doctor by also as a patient how Upper Cervical treatment really does work.

CHAPTER 9

A Short History

Chiropractic is specific, or it is nothing.

Dr BJ Palmer

―――――――――

Before we proceed, it may be worth looking back through the history of Upper Cervical care to discover where these problems of ignorance, prejudice and superstition originated in the first place.

―――――――――

The Founder

The history of Upper Cervical begins with the origins of chiropractic itself in 1895.

In a small office building in Davenport, Iowa, a young man named Daniel David (DD) Palmer worked as a magnetic healer. Also working in this building as a janitor was a man named Harvey Lillard, whom DD Palmer noticed had a very prominent protrusion on his neck. After some discussion, Palmer convinced Mr Lillard to allow him to manipulate this particular vertebra to see what affect it would have.

Even to Palmer, the outcome of this event was completely unexpected, for Harvey Lillard, whose hearing had been severely impaired for over 17 years could suddenly hear again! [cxviii]

DD Palmer was fascinated how the correction of a vertebral misalignment could cause such an astonishing result.

Even in 1895, it was already a well-established medical fact that the spinal cord was the communication link between the brain and the body. Palmer extrapolated that a spinal subluxation had the potential to disrupt the transmission of nerve impulses, and that this interference could inhibit the body's innate ability to heal itself. He reasoned further that this type of system malfunction could manifest as pain, dysfunction and disease anywhere in the body.

He concluded that his discovery of chiropractic (a term coined by one of DD Palmer's patients, Reverend Samuel Weed) could restore the proper function of the spinal cord, restore the innate healing mechanisms of the body, and therefore restore the health and vitality of the human body.

Originally DD Palmer wanted to keep his discovery a secret. However, several individuals including his only son Bartlett Joshua (BJ) would eventually convince him otherwise. Two years after his discovery in 1897, DD Palmer would found the Palmer School of Chiropractic. Five years later in 1902, the first class of 15 students would graduate.

These first chiropractors included notable physicians, surgeons, homeopaths, and also BJ Palmer himself, whose rise within the chiropractic profession a few years later would mark the birth of Upper Cervical. [cxix]

The Developer

The relationship between father and son was tenuous at the best of times, but especially so after BJ persuaded DD to sell the school and its assets to him in 1906. [cxx]

One of the most divisive issues between the two was their vision for the young profession.

DD Palmer practiced full-spinal specific treatment and developed the Metric system of adjusting. The Metric system dictated that a chiropractor adjust the spine when there was a symptomatic complaint associated with a specific vertebra. For example, if a person described lower back pain and kidney problems, the chiropractor would adjust the 12th thoracic vertebra (T12).

The style of spinal manipulation taught by DD Palmer—that is, to adjust the most palpable vertebra that correlates with the location of symptoms—remains the basis for many general chiropractors even today.

On the other side, BJ Palmer believed that this form of spinal manipulation did not address many people's underlying issues. Initially he did practice the same Metric style as his father. However, he recognized quickly that the most remarkable episodes of chiropractic healing occurred with upper cervical spinal treatment.

With BJ Palmer at the helm of the Palmer School, he would begin to narrow his focus increasingly toward the upper cervical spine. In 1909, he incorporated x-ray (itself only in existence since 1895) into the school curriculum and developed the practice of spinography, a method to see the exact nature of a subluxation in order to determine the best angle of correction. [cxxi]

After years of research in 1930, BJ Palmer introduced the "Hole in One" (HIO) method—the first Upper Cervical specific chiropractic adjustment. [cxxii]

The original HIO procedure used a knee-chest style table where patients would kneel on a small riser with their heads rested on a firm headpiece. The chiropractor would then place his palm over the atlas, and then deliver a high-velocity, low amplitude (HVLA) downward force at the exact angle that was measured from the Upper Cervical x-rays.

Dr Palmer would continue to refine his HIO method to include a mechanical drop-piece, which allowed for a sharper yet softer correction.

In 1935, BJ would established the Palmer Research Clinic, a state-of-the-art, world renowned centre, which included a huge number of facilities: an x-ray department complete with fluoroscopy (moving and 3D x-rays); on-site pathology, urinalysis and instrumentation labs, which included precursors to modern ECG and EEG machines; an exercise and rehabilitation department; and a luxurious recovery garden. The clinic employed not only Upper Cervical chiropractors, but also medical doctors and researchers. cxxiii

BJ Palmer believed firmly that the precise correction of the upper cervical subluxation was the key to good health. He also believed that it was this one thing that distinguished chiropractic from osteopathy and other forms of spinal manipulation.

He so firmly believed it that Upper Cervical care was the only style of chiropractic instructed at the Palmer School for the next 30 years until his death in 1961.

———————

While BJ Palmer was a dynamic force for chiropractic in the early 20th Century, it did not mean that the entire profession was united behind him. Across America and throughout the world, new colleges with different values would rise. Many of these schools were heavily influenced by the methods taught by DD Palmer and also by Dr Andrew Still, the founder of osteopathy. Other chiropractic innovators such as Clarence Gonstead, Clay Thompson, Hugh Logan and Major DeJarnette also worked beyond the influence of the Palmer School to develop many of the chiropractic methods that exist today.

Although BJ Palmer and Upper Cervical care dominated the chiropractic landscape for the early 20th Century, the tides of chiropractic would shift again as Dr Palmer 's son, David assumed leadership of the profession.

———————

The Educator

As a child and young man, David Palmer lived much of his personal and professional life in the shadow of his father. Although BJ Palmer was certainly a dynamic leader, he lacked financial prudence. Repeatedly, his escapades and indulgences would bring the Palmer School to the edge of financial oblivion.

With an education in both business and chiropractic, David Palmer saw that radical change was necessary to elevate chiropractic as a respectable profession and the Palmer School as a viable institution.

His solution was to transform the Palmer School into a fully accredited university.

Symbolic of the many changes that he would make, David Palmer started by erasing thousands of inspirational epigrams that his father had written across the walls of the school. The Palmer Research Clinic was cleared, all its records archived (or destroyed) and un-published, and a new teaching clinic was established.

Most significantly, full-spinal adjusting techniques were also re-introduced into the curriculum. It was the Upper Cervical courses that were sacrificed to make room.

Few would argue that the changes instituted by David Palmer were necessary. Like the fiery death of a phoenix before its glorious rebirth, these changes allowed the school to be reborn as Palmer College of Chiropractic, an esteemed institute on par with any medical or professional university in the world.

As David Palmer would remark, "Palmer is to chiropractic is what Sterling is to silver."

At the same time, it may be argued that part of the school's original identity was lost. Upper Cervical care remains a core study at Palmer even today, and it does maintain a strong following. However, it is now regarded by many chiropractors as a historical or elective study rather than the first-choice method of chiropractic treatment.

To compound the problem, the division between DD and BJ Palmer remains to this day (old feelings die hard!). Although there are dozens of chiropractic programs throughout the world, Upper Cervical is an advanced study in only four of them: 3 in America and 1 in New Zealand.

That is the reason that most people including many chiropractors have never heard of Upper Cervical. Simply put, they don't know it exists.

CHAPTER 10

Upper Cervical Evolution

Those who cannot remember the past are condemned to repeat it.

George Santayana

Although Upper Cervical care seemed doomed for oblivion, the tireless efforts of many doctors including the former patients and students of BJ Palmer has allowed Upper Cervical care to survive, evolve and enter its second renaissance in the 21st Century.

One of these most influential Upper Cervical pioneers was Dr John F Grostic. As a young man, Grostic was diagnosed with terminal Hodgkin's disease (aka leukemia). In desperation, his family turned to Dr BJ Palmer, who had only recently introduced his HIO method. Against all odds, Grostic made a remarkable recovery in just a few weeks. [cxxiv]

Three years later, Dr Grostic would graduate as a chiropractor from the Palmer School and dedicate his life to the advancement of Upper Cervical care.

With the Palmer School over 500km (300+ miles) from his hometown in Michigan, Dr Grostic continued to receive Upper Cervical care from his local chiropractor. However, Grostic noted his local chiropractor was not able to reproduce Dr Palmer 's adjustment, which would resolve his condition for weeks at a time instead of just a few days.

Discussing this matter with BJ Palmer on several occasions, Dr Grostic came to realise that Dr Palmer was performing customised HIO corrections.

The HIO method could only describe the relative direction of a subluxation: for example, "PRI" which would mean that the vertebra was misaligned in a posterior (back), right and inferior (down) direction.

Customization was not a formal part of the HIO method. Nevertheless, that was exactly what Dr Palmer was doing. It was a problem that he posed in his book, *The Subluxation Specific-The Adjustment Specific*. "Should I list the adjustment P x R xx I xxx, it would say that it should be adjusted P, but the adjustment should be TWICE AS MUCH from the 'R' as from 'P' and three times as much from 'I.'" [cxxv]

By studying upper cervical biomechanics and by applying principles of mechanical engineering, Dr Grostic sought to resolve this problem. In 1939, he formally introduced a new Upper Cervical method that could express an adjustment vector in mathematical terms.

The result was an adjustment that could be customized and reproduced for each-and-every patient.

Dr Grostic also developed a more accurate system to measure the atlas misalignment on x-ray, and he refined the adjustment procedure itself so that an Upper Cervical chiropractor could perform it by hand or with a mechanical instrument. [cxxvi]

After Dr Grostic's death in 1964, his son Dr John D Grostic would continue his father 's work, which today is known as Orthospinology. [cxxvii]

Case Report: Emily's Story (Part I)

Of all the remarkable episodes of healing I have seen, there are two that stand out among the others.

The first is Joe's story, which I have already started to tell in this book.

The second is Emily's story. Emily was a bright and gifted child with an abundance of energy, who was referred to me by a former colleague. She had travelled over 1000km (600 miles) with her mother Christine, who was desperate to help her 10-year old daughter.

Although I knew that Emily would arrive with some type of severe condition, I never would have suspected that she would come to me bound in a wheelchair and unable to walk.

Even then, I did not appreciate the full extent of her problem until she crawled from her wheelchair to sit on my examination table. I have seen many people with acute lower back pain, who are unable to stand upright or even move. However, Emily's problem was immeasurably worse.

It was like someone had broken her body in half, pulled her torso sideways, twisted her spine 90 degrees, and then fused her back together. Every muscle from the top of her neck to the bottom of her feet was locked in a spasm.

Worse yet, Emily could feel every terrible sensation as if her own body was tearing her apart.

"Six months ago she was completely fine," Christine started to tell me. "Nothing was wrong with her. She was playing her violin, running around, going to school and doing all the things kids are supposed to do.

"The only thing we noticed at first was that she was walking funny. Her feet were pointed sideways like a duck. But Emily used to walk on her toes when she was younger. We thought it was just a phase like that. So did our doctor."

"Yeah," Emily chimed in. "But he said the same thing even when my back was popping."

"'Popping?'" I asked.

"My back was popping," Emily repeated as she clicked her tongue a few times.

"And it was loud," Christine added. "I could hear it from our living room even if she was walking down the hall,"

I had to admit that I was puzzled. I knew of many clicking sounds that can come from the body: joint cavitation, which is the clicking sound associated with spinal manipulation; tendons rubbing against each other; ligaments tearing; and even bones breaking. What Christine and Emily were describing seemed to be something different. Fortunately,

Christine had recorded a video clip, which she proceeded to show me.

"This was four months ago."

The video started with Emily facing away from the camera and slouched forward. As Emily stood upright, I could see a spastic twitch in her lower back followed with a sharp popping sound. It sounded like the noise a ping-pong ball makes when you bounce it off a concrete floor.

Seeing this video, I realised that the most likely source of the sound was a tendon in Emily's lower back snapping over a bone. Why it was doing that, I still had no idea.

"It did that for about a month," Christine said, "but then it just stopped.

Emily rejoined the conversation. "But my back was really hurting. We went to the chiropractors and physiotherapists in town, but all they did was massage and crack my back, which really hurt."

"We tried an acupuncturist too," Christine added, "but that didn't help much either." She then showed me a second video. "This was three months ago."

The video showed Emily trying to walk up a flight of stairs with her school bag dragging behind her. Just as they had described Emily's feet were pointing outward rather markedly. However, the more noticeable problems were that her knees were angled sharply inward, that she was bent sideways and also that she was hunched forward.

"Things just kept getting worse from there," Christine continued trying to hold back her tears. "We've been to all the specialists back home, and they don't know what's wrong. Now we've been to all the specialists in the city. They don't know what's wrong either."

"I hate hospitals," Emily added with a grimace.

"We've taken her for x-rays, bone scans, tests where they put needles into her arms, legs and back [NCV, aka Nerve Conduction Velocity tests, which test for neurological disease], CTs and MRIs of her full spine and head. She's even had a PET scan, but they still can't find what's wrong with her.

"The only thing they've given her are muscle relaxants, which just make her drowsy. Plus she has a back brace."

Christine lifted Emily's shirt to reveal a plastic corset-like cast that was holding her spine in place.

"It digs into my skin," Emily said.

"They've said if she keeps getting worse they're going to put rods into her spine. But they don't know if even that will help."

At this point, Christine's tears were flowing freely.

"What I don't understand is how this can happen so quickly to a healthy girl. And why no one can tell us what's wrong with her.

"We're here because we've heard about this atlas treatment. We've tried everything else, and we don't know what else to do."

I cannot begin to imagine the nightmare that Christine was suffering as she watched helplessly as her little girl's health progressively deteriorated in such a short period for no explicable reason.

For me, it was heart-wrenching to watch those videos knowing that only six months ago Emily had been completely normal. I had no idea what I could possibly say or do to help ease their pain.

The only thing that I did know was that I would do everything I could to help them.

(Continued in Chapter 14)

<hr>

The Next Generation

The Grostic procedure would give rise to two sibling techniques: NUCCA and Atlas Orthogonality. Dr Ralph Gregory refined the manual adjusting aspects of the Grostic method, and in 1966 he introduced the National Upper Cervical Chiropractic Association (NUCCA) procedure. [cxxviii] Dr Roy Sweat refined the instrument adjusting aspects, and in 1981 he introduced Atlas Orthogonality (AO) and a system to measure an upper cervical alignment in degrees. [cxxix] Atlas Orthogonal itself has evolved with the advent of

Advanced Orthogonal introduced in 2007 by Drs Stan Pierce Senior and Junior. [cxxx]

Equally notable are the achievements of numerous other Upper Cervical doctors, whose procedures evolved directly from BJ Palmer's HIO method (today known as Toggle Recoil).

As Dr Palmer came to favour the drop-piece mechanism and the Toggle Recoil style of upper cervical adjusting, Dr Michael Kale continued with the original knee-chest style of adjusting, which he believed allowed for a more effective correction. In 1964 he introduced the Kale method, which through the efforts of Dr Robert Kessinger continues today as Upper Cervical Knee Chest Specific (UCKCS). [cxxxi]

Dr William Blair pioneered the use of stereoscopic x-ray in order to measure joint asymmetry that may otherwise reduce the effectiveness of the correction. He also developed a unique x-ray system in order to see in perfect detail the true nature of an upper cervical misalignment. In 1951 he introduced the Blair method of upper cervical adjusting. [cxxxii]

These six methods—Toggle Recoil, Orthospinology, NUCCA, Atlas Orthogonal, Kale and Blair—account for the vast majority of the techniques used by Upper Cervical chiropractors today.

Although there are differences among these techniques, they share the common aim to correct an atlas subluxation in the most precise way possible.

No method is more effective than any other, and each one helped to create life-changing results for people all around the world.

As true today as when BJ Palmer recognized it a century ago, most of the incredible anecdotes, case studies and reports of chiropractic healing have involved the upper cervical spine.

Make no mistake about it—Upper Cervical treatment is not the same as general spinal manipulation. Those differences will be elaborated further in later chapters. Until then, I hope that this tangent into the history of Upper Cervical care may explain why it remains one of the best-kept secrets in healthcare.

Ignorance, prejudice and superstition will always exist. However, the solution to overcome these enemies is as it always has been: knowledge. Knowledge that there is another way. And that it has a century of practice, research and refinement behind it!

I believe it is now time to return to Joe's story and to the moments that I decided to lay aside my own superstitions in order to help him as best as I could.

CHAPTER 11

The Original Injury

Natural forces within us are the true healers of disease.

Hippocrates

—————————

What have I gotten myself into?

I hurried down the stairs into the clinic basement where the radiology department was located.

Over the past three months, the Palmer clinic had received several major upgrades. In fact, the clinic was an entirely new building complete with millions of dollars of state-of-the-art equipment.

The changes were most evident in the x-ray department. Gone were the days working in tiny dark rooms with chemicals and wet films. Now were the days working in bright open spaces with computer processors and digital cassettes.

The new clinic was absolutely marvelous. The only problem was that it wasn't working yet. The transition between the old and new Palmer clinics was far from a seamless process.

As just one example, when you needed a patient's file, you could never find it.

Even if you found it, then you would have to setup a new computer file to use from that date onward.

Even if you setup that file, then you would have to navigate through the most horrible, unfriendly software to write even a one-line note.

And even if you figured out how to use the software, the clinic administrators would decide that they wanted you to write your notes a different way... which meant that you would have to start the whole process again!

Neither the doctors nor the interns knew what was happening from one day to the next. As often happens in the comedy of life, you embrace the madness and soldier-on in spite of it all.

The administrators would eventually get the clinic systems working efficiently (after I graduated, of course). From what I hear, the Palmer Chiropractic Clinic now uses some of the most sophisticated hardware and software in the world. It was just a shame that my class were the guinea pigs that helped make it happen.

For all the craziness that was already happening that morning, my only hope was that things would not get any worse in the x-ray department.

Louise was the head radiologist on duty that morning. Although I had finished my final shift as a blue coat and had retired a week earlier, I hoped that she would be able to help me one last time.

"Shouldn't you be relaxing on your day off?" Louise teased with a smile.

"I thought so too, but apparently I'm not any good at it."

Louise listened empathetically as I explained the situation. It took her only a couple of seconds to contemplate before she replied calmly, "Yes, I think we can manage that."

Yes. Finally some good news!

"There may be just a few problems though," she added.

The first problem was that we could use only the general x-ray equipment. All the Upper Cervical x-ray equipment was still in the old clinic across the street, and Joe was in absolutely no condition to make that trip.

The second problem was that the software required to analyze the digital x-ray images was still not installed on any of the clinic computers. Even if we were able to take the x-rays, we would still have no proper way to analyze them.

Fortunately, I had solutions for these two potential dilemmas.

When I was on shift with Louise, she had allowed me to experiment with alternate ways to take Upper Cervical x-rays using standard radiographic equipment. As an intern with too much time on his hands, I had also experimented with ways to analyze those x-rays on the computer using simple lines, point measurements and hand calculations.

Although these methods were not ideal, they still achieved good results. More importantly, they allowed the Upper Cervical staff doctors and interns to keep working when everyone else in the clinic had no idea how to do anything.

As I described my plan for Louise, I realised suddenly why my dad needed me to help him with Joe. I was the only person in the clinic who knew how to take the modified Upper Cervical x-rays and who understood the clinic computer software well enough to analyze them.

There were two more problems that Louise and I foresaw, and both of them were administrative ones.

Like any other institution, the clinic had regulations that all interns were required to follow. In order to schedule an x-ray appointment, interns required a signed report from a staff doctor to prove that there was a legitimate reason to take x-rays in the first place.

Of course, I didn't have that.

To complicate matters, Joe was technically a patient of the student teaching clinic across the street. Therefore, he should not have been admitted into the main clinic to see my dad in the first place. Additionally, to transfer his file for even a single treatment would have been an extremely complicated task that would have taken all day.

From a strict legal point of view, we were caught in limbo.

Fortunately, Louise had solutions for these two problems. She had worked with my dad for over 10 years. I can only assume that she must have sensed that he never would have made such an unusual request unless it was really urgent.

"Well, I think I can make an exception for Dr Hannah this time. As long as your dad has all the paperwork when your patient arrives, we'll be fine. I'll just put his name on the schedule in the student clinic, but then we'll just take the x-rays here."

More good news!

"Thanks, Louise. You're the best."

"I know," she responded with another smile. "The only opening I have this morning is in 10 minutes. Do you think you can have your patient ready by then?"

He has an appointment! The hard part is already over!

A heavy dose of reality set in when I remembered that Joe could not stand on his own, let alone walk. Somehow we would have to get him downstairs. On top of that, we had only 10 minutes to complete a stack of paperwork that would normally take 30 minutes.

"No," I replied hurrying back up the stairs. "But I'll do the best I can."

———

Throughout this book I have used the terms signs and symptoms. Before we go much further, I think it is the proper time to define the difference between them.

A sign is something that an outside person can see or measure about you. Common examples are temperature, the colour of your eyes, bony prominences in your neck, and your posture (e.g., the straightness of your head).

A symptom is something that only you can feel: coldness or warmness, itchiness in your eyes, soreness in your neck or any other sensation you may experience (e.g., the heaviness of your head).

The cause of an upper cervical subluxation is a simple yet complex topic.

On one hand, there is only one thing that can cause an atlas misalignment: trauma to the head or neck. [cxxxiii] [cxxxiv] On the other hand, if that primary subluxation remains uncorrected for a long time, the more complex the problem becomes.

A Simple Explanation

Dr Julie Mayer Hunt gives the following analogy.

"Stack up 24 dominoes [and] put a bowling ball on top. Biomechanically that's the structure we're working with. And the critical area is right there at the base of the skull. If you look at the way that it's designed and put together, [the atlas] is the critical area that will discern where the weight of the head is being carried. And if you centre that, the rest of the spine can balance with it." [cxxxv]

Dr Tom Forest elaborates further.

"The spine from the low back all the way up to the mid- neck region has interlocking joints that limit how far the bones can move. But ironically enough the atlas and axis, the top two are not shaped the same way. They don't have the same bony locks. The segments are held in place by muscles and ligaments. So as a result it's a more unstable area. And that's of course what gives us the tremendous amount of mobility we have in the neck area.

"The problem is that with that increased mobility, it makes us more susceptible to injury in that area." [cxxxvi]

In simplest terms, therefore, it is the atlas that is most likely to be affected if you suffer a head or neck injury.

There are two types of trauma that can cause a subluxation:

- specific trauma; and
- repetitive trauma.

Specific trauma refers to one or more memorable events that cause significant damage to your neck. Some examples include things like motor vehicle accidents, head-to- head sport collisions, landing on your head after a fall, or other violent whiplash-like injuries.

No less significant are minor things like getting hit in the head by a football, riding a roller coaster, or falling off a snow, surf or skateboard.

Repetitive trauma refers to habitual activities that cause micro-damage to your neck. Like continuously stretching a rubber band to its breaking point, any activity repeated enough times will accumulative damage just as significant as if it was caused from a specific event.

Some examples include things like sleeping face down on your stomach, watching television with your head propped on the edge of a couch, working on a computer or talking on the phone.

———

Many Upper Cervical chiropractors look to childhood as the time of the first subluxation.

Although this statement may sound incredible, consider it fully before rushing to judgment.

Remember the reckless joy of being a child. Children fly off furniture, jump off trampolines and run headfirst into anything they stumble across. Then they cry for five minutes, bounce up and do it all over again. No less jarring are the numerous tumbles, knocks and falls that children experience when learning to crawl, stand, walk and ride bicycles.

By the age of two, a child's head is already 3.0-3.5 Kg, which is approximately 25% its total body weight and already 60% of its total adult size. [cxxxvii] [cxxxviii]

The concern is that the soft tissues and bones of a two-year old are nowhere near as strong as they are in an adult. As a result, even a very minor injury like bumping into the edge of a coffee table may be enough to cause the atlas imbalance.

A subluxation may even happen during birth itself. Good obstetricians take the utmost care to ensure that the birthing process is safe for both mum and bub. However, that does not always mean that everything goes according to plan.

Difficult births, breach presentations and entangled cords are all potential sources of injury and trauma that may cause a spinal misalignment even before a newborn baby has the chance to take its first breath. [cxxxix] [cxl]

In no way do I mean that parents should be fearful or should rush their children to a pediatrician or chiropractor whenever they take a tumble. Instead, I advocate common sense and vigilance.

When it comes to parenting, trust your intuition. If you have a gut feeling that something is wrong with your child, or if you notice any significant change with your child's behaviour, then it is worth getting a professional opinion.

CHAPTER 12

The First Sign

*The doctor of the future will give no medicine, but
will instruct his patient in the care of the human
frame, in diet and in the cause and
prevention of disease.*

Thomas Edison

Many people do not recognize the early signs that they may have
an atlas problem.

When an injury happens, many people do not notice any initial
symptoms at all. Many people also assume that if they experience
symptoms that resolve quickly that they must be okay. Hence, they
go on with normal life as if nothing ever happened.

If you were to suffer a car accident today, you may not experience any muscle soreness until a week from now. You may not

experience headaches or acute backaches until you start a new job five years from now. And you may not suffer arthritis or dizziness for another 15-20 years. [cxli]

Your body is so amazing in its ability to adapt to injury and stress that it may take weeks, months or even years before any hint of a problem erupts from beneath the surface.

For that reason it is important to remember that just because you think that you "feel well" does not always mean that everything is okay.

———————

Poor posture or body imbalance (see Chapter 5) is often the earliest sign of an atlas subluxation.

Posture may be the result of an abnormal bony development: for example, scoliosis or Scheuermann's disease, two spinal conditions that cause excessive curving of the spine. Poor posture may also be the result of simple laziness.

Yes, children sit too long at school desks, watch too much television and play too many contact sports. Just as well, adults sit too long at computers, spend too much time commuting and then do too much repetitive labour but not enough exercise to maintain their core strength.

However, postural problems are most often the manifestation of an upper cervical subluxation.

Imagine that you build a crooked house. No matter how much aesthetic work you do to make it appear straighter, the simple fact will remain that the house is crooked.

The same is true with your body. If you have a subluxation that makes your body crooked, no matter how many exercises you do—no matter how many times you are told to stop slouching and stand straight—your body will remain crooked.

The only way to correct the structural imbalance is to correct the cause of the imbalance in the first place. And there is not a drug or exercise in the world that will correct a subluxated vertebra.

———————

Scoliosis Neurosis

I have a particular hang-up when doctors use the term scoliosis to describe what should be called a lateral spinal curvature.

Studies have demonstrated that people who have been diagnosed with scoliosis have markedly poor self-esteem and body image perceptions. [cxlii] It is almost as if scoliosis is perceived to be just as severe as something like terminal cancer.

It is more than just semantics: scoliosis is not the same as a spinal curvature.

To diagnose scoliosis requires that the angle of the spinal curve is measured to be at least 10 degrees from normal (more appropriately at least 20 degrees). [cxliii]

My neurosis stems from numerous instances that I have tried to explain to people, who have a 5 degree curve on their x-rays that they do not have a spinal scoliosis and that they do not have a dangerous condition that will cripple them for life.

More often than not, lateral spinal curves are nothing more than body imbalance, and if you correct the cause of the imbalance at the atlas and axis, the problem disappears on its own.

Even if a true scoliosis is present, it may still be related to an upper cervical subluxation. I have seen many cases first- hand of idiopathic or physiological scoliosis where curves in excess of 30 degrees have improved just by correcting the alignment of the atlas.

In truth, I do not expect the medical or chiropractic communities to change their language any time in the near future. It is my hope instead that this message reaches the people, who need to hear it most.

I also hope that these people realise that Upper Cervical care may be able to help whether their problem is scoliosis or just a lateral spinal curve.

───────────

Imagine that a 4-year old girl is trying to get her mother 's attention. She starts tugging on her mother 's clothing, softly repeating, "Mum ... Mum ... Mum." If mum pays no attention to her daughter 's pleading, the young girl only tugs harder and shouts louder, "Mum! ... Mum! ... Mum!!" Eventually, mum will not be able to ignore the pleading, and in order to preserve her sanity she will have to drop whatever she is doing and pay attention.

The human body works the same way. The initial postural signs that a problem is present may be mute. Given enough time your body will start to talk to you: first with a whisper and then with a normal voice. However, if you ignore that voice, your body will resort to yelling at you (pain!) until you are fully conscious of the problem and finally do something about it.

Of those early symptoms or "whispers," you may experience random aches, minor niggles or vague twinges. You have an "off day" where you do not feel like your normal, pleasant self. You may even have nothing more than an intuitive feeling that something is wrong.

In short, you may just not feel well. The problem can be even more difficult to identify with children.

Children may experience headaches, recurrent ear infections, fevers or chronic illness. They are more likely to be lethargic, fussy or colicky. [cxliv cxlv cxlvi] They are equally likely to be hyperactive, irritable or inattentive. However, they may only say something so simple as, "I don't feel good."

It's Just a Headache

There is no such a thing as a normal headache.

There is an older but extremely interesting report from 1970 that deserves attention. Medical physicians Dr Murray Braaf and Dr Samual Rosner considered over 5000 headache cases over their 20-year careers. They noted the following:

"Many chronic headache sufferers date their headaches back to their childhood. Most of these unfortunates have been examined and re-examined through the years in medical centres and by private physicians. Since no definite cause has been discovered, the headaches were usually treated through the use of psychiatry. They would try teaching the patient to live with the pain."

It was their conclusion that was most interesting.

"More than 90% of recurring headaches can be traced to mechanical derangement of the cervical or neck portion of the spine produced by an injury." [cxlvii]

Many other things do contribute toward headaches: e.g., hormone changes, food additives, industrial chemicals and allergies. It is interesting that even these cases may have an underlying vertebral subluxation, which contributes toward the problem.

Considering that 90% of all headaches may be related to a neck misalignment, it would be far better for people to learn that an Upper Cervical chiropractor may be the best person to fix the problem.

So why people believe it is okay to, "Just take an aspirin to stop the pain because it's just a headache," is beyond me.

An atlas subluxation is caused by trauma to the head and neck. That trauma may happen during adulthood but is more likely during childhood.

The early signs are usually postural problems such as body imbalance. If the problem is not corrected and enough time allowed to pass, other symptoms will be certain to appear.

That is the simple explanation.

However, it only applies with the first subluxation. In the next chapter, I will describe what happens thereafter and how a simple problem with a simple solution becomes so complex and difficult to manage.

CHAPTER 13

Too Much Stress

The cause of subluxation is trauma, poison, or auto-suggestion.

DD Palmer

A little out of breath, I relayed the message from Louise to my dad. As tight as it would be to get everything ready in just 10 minutes, we really had no other choice. Without wasting any time, we made a split decision: Dr Hannah and Rob would complete the paperwork; Kevin and I would help Joe get downstairs.

Exactly how we were going to do that I had no idea.

Kevin and I popped back into Joe's dark room and explained the plan to him.

"If Kevin and I help you, do you think you can walk?"

"I'll make it," he responded with admirable determination.

"There is an elevator just around the corner. The x-ray rooms are right at the bottom. We'll hold your weight, and we'll go at your pace. If you keep your eyes closed and just put one foot in front of the other, we should be okay."

We gave Joe a moment to summon his strength. When he was ready, Kevin and I helped him into a sitting position, wrapped his arms over our shoulders and then slowly pulled him to his feet.

Step by step, the three of us shuffled through the clinic toward the elevator. Seeing the solemn expressions on the faces of other interns as we passed by, it felt like we were carrying a wounded soldier off the battlefield. Step by step, we marched on.

The elevator ride to the radiology department went smoothly, and Louise was there at the bottom to greet us. She directed us straight into the x-ray room, where she had already dimmed the lights and prepared a chair for Joe.

Although we arrived in one piece, the trip had taken its toll on Joe. He collapsed into the chair as if he had been walking for days. The trip had been less than five minutes.

"Joe, will you be okay if I get a few things ready while we wait for Dr Hannah?"

"Yes. Thank you."

"I'll stay with him until you guys are ready," Kevin added.

I have great respect for Kevin, whose caring attitude and support went a long way that morning. We all know people for whom we would do anything to help if they ever needed it.

Few of us are ever called into action like Kevin was. If not for him, I have no idea how Joe would have managed.

Just as I joined Louise in the waiting area, Dr Hannah and Rob arrived. Louise checked that their paperwork was all in order.

"Looks good to me," she informed us. "You can start whenever you're ready."

Poor Rob. Despite his best attempts to conceal his nervousness, his pale skin and nervous eyes gave him away. All Palmer interns learn about Upper Cervical x-rays, but only those of us who studied the advanced methods actually learn how to take them.

He was in way over his head.

"Don't worry," I assured him. "That's why I'm here."

I explained that I would be doing the actual x-ray setups but that he would receive the official credit for pushing the exposure button. "Piggyback" was the term that we used at Palmer to describe this sort of arrangement, and it was quite a common practice.

In short, piggy-backing meant that I would do the physical work but that Rob would have to do all paperwork afterwards. I still believe that I got the better end of the deal!

At last, we were ready to start. All I needed to do was explain a few final things for Joe.

"We're going to do five x-rays, "I said. "I need you to be able to hold your head up straight. Whatever feels most normal and most comfortable for you. I know it's really hard for you to hold your head up, but can you do that?"

"Yes. Thank you."

"Okay, good. I'll give you a moment to rest between each x-ray. I'll still do each one as fast as I can. If you need to rest, let me know as well.

"Do what you have to do. I'll be okay."

"I may have to shine a light in your eyes a bit so that I can do the setup properly. You can keep them closed, and I'll warn you before I do it. Are you ready Joe?"

"Let's do it. Thank you."

With his vote of confidence, we started.

Your body has the innate ability to heal itself. If you slice your finger on a sharp knife, the wound will heal itself. If you break your forearm, the bones will heal without outside intervention.

Whether it heals the right way or the wrong way is another matter.

With a broken bone, you have a few hours or sometimes even a few days to see an orthopedist, who can prepare a cast so that your forearm will heal properly. If on the other hand (no pun intended) you do not see an orthopedist your forearm does not heal properly, you may lose the ability to twist your wrist.

Remember that the orthopedist does not cause your forearm to heal. The orthopedist can only facilitate the healing process.

Likewise, an Upper Cervical chiropractor does not cause your spine to heal either. The doctor can only facilitate the healing process. The problem is a perception of urgency: that is, people have a great sense of urgency if they suffer a broken bone but not if they misalign an atlas vertebra!

Because the initial signs of a subluxation are so subtle, many people do not seek the expertise of an Upper Cervical doctor for weeks, months or years after the injury. The result may be that the body has healed improperly.

Thus, what was once a relatively simple injury with a simple solution is now a complex problem that may require extensive treatment to correct.

It is my unfortunate duty to warn you that the following chapters contain some heavy-duty science stuff. If it were not critically important in order to understand how upper cervical problems become complex, I would cut it in a heartbeat.

Needless to say, it is that important.

With my sincerest apologies, shall we get on with it?

The Language of the Human Body

The nervous system speaks only one language, which is the language of neurotransmitters. Neurotransmitters are molecules that are synthesized and released from neurons. Some common neurotransmitters include dopamine, serotonin, acetylcholine, substance P and epinephrine.

Like letters of the alphabet, over 100 different neurotransmitters interact with other neurons to convey specific messages along the nervous system. From the brain to the body, messages are send downward so that the muscles, organs and other tissues will function properly.

From the body to the brain, messages are sent upward so that the brain can assemble these letters into meaningful words and sentences. These types of ascending messages originate from thousands of specialized neuron sensors located throughout the body.

The function of these sensors is to send a continuous stream of information to the brain about the body's internal and external environment.

Some sensors detect wave frequencies that are interpreted in the brain as physical vibration, sound and sight. Other sensors detect physical sensations such as touch, movement and physical damage (aka nociception), which are interpreted in the brain as pain.

Physical receptors also provide the brain with information about muscle tone and body position (i.e., proprioception).

Other sensors monitor the body's internal chemical environment: for example, blood acidity, vitamin and mineral levels, and oxygen concentrations. Chemical receptors also receive information from the external environment, which correspond to the odour and taste of foods, fluids and other substances.

The point I would like to make is that it does not matter if a sensor detects a physical, chemical or emotional stimulus. All stimuli are translated into the same language: i.e., the language of neurotransmitters.

Shortly we will discuss the various stimuli that can aggravate an upper cervical problem. First, we will consider two reasons from a neurophysiological perspective that the problem becomes so complex: muscle memory and structural mal-adaptation.

Muscle Memory

If you have been told thousands of times since you were a child that, "You're stupid," you may believe it is true. From a neurological perspective, muscle memory is no different.

Muscle memory is a form of neurological learning through motor repetition.

Think of an activity that requires great coordination and focus when you learn how to do it. The classic example is learning to ride a bicycle. Never mind things like controlling your speed, minding your surroundings and looking our for other hazards on the road: the first time you hopped on a bike you probably had to focus all your attention just to keep your balance!

Fast forward to the present day. Even if you have not been on a bicycle in years, you would probably be able to ride without a moment's hesitation.

That is muscle memory. In truth, it is actually neurological memory, which coordinates your muscles to work in an automatic, unconscious manner.

Muscle memory includes any activity where the saying, "Practice makes perfect," applies. It also includes anything that "You could do with your eyes closed," like typing on a computer keyboard, playing a musical instrument, doing a professional trade and so forth.

Muscle memory also includes the tone of your muscles and the position of joints within your body. Were you ever told as a child, "Don't make faces or it will stay that way?" There is some truth in that saying.

If your body becomes habituated to being stuck in a certain position, then it may stay that way!

Two things may be worth consideration at this point.

First, should you try to adopt new muscle patterns such as sitting upright, walking lighter or moving your neck differently, you may find it extremely difficult to break your old muscle memory patterns.

Second, should any stimulus activate the centres of the brain responsible for old muscle memory patterns, your body may assume the old motor pattern and reignite symptoms associated with an old injury.

Let me give an example. When I first moved to Australia I slept on a futon mattress. Although it wasn't the most comfortable thing in the world, it did serve its purpose. Plus it was the only thing that I could afford.

For the first few months I was able to get a decent night of sleep. After 6 months, however, I would wake every morning with lower back pain. Eventually I would save up, wise up and buy a proper bed. Sure enough, my back problems disappeared within a few days.

Several months later my parents came out of Australia for a brief stay, and I offered them my bed. Thinking nothing of it, I decided to sleep on the futon. After just one night, my back was as sore as it had been all those months ago.

Although I did not have a severe injury, the stimulus of sleeping on that futon was sufficient to trigger the old neurological pathways and muscle memories associated with my lower back pain.

I share this story to illustrate how muscle memory works and also to show how it may relate to chronic pain and health problems. Like WL Bateman says, "If you keep on doing what you've always done, you'll keep on getting what you've always got."

———

Structural Mal-adaptation

The other reason that an injury becomes chronic has to do with a process known as structural mal-adaptation.

Think of the difference in body type between an Olympic swimmer and a rugby player. Neither physique is better than the other, but through sport-specific training each athlete is better adapted to excel in his respective sport. Although the rugby player will not be as agile through the water, the swimmer will not be as powerful on the field.

Structural adaptation, otherwise known as the Wolff- Davis law, is the process by which muscles, ligaments and bones can be re-shaped over time.

Your body is structurally dynamic. It continually remodels itself in accordance with the activities that you perform every day. Structural adaption only becomes a problem when your body adapts to chronic pathological stress (or even worse, it adapts to not moving at all).

To paraphrase the old sports adage, "If you abuse it or don't use it, you lose it."

The consequence of such abuse is known as neuromusculoskeletal mal-adaptation, or simply mal- adaptation for our purposes).

Imagine that you have a leaky roof. As a quick remedy, you toss a bucket on the floor and throw a tarp over the roof. Although this patch may work as a short-term solution, it does not fix the problem. In fact, it may only make things worse if the tarp disperses the water and creates a bigger hole.

Think of your body as a machine. If you follow the instructions in the operations manual and take proper care of the machine, it will remain in fine condition for many years. However, if you don't follow the manual, abuse the machine or do not service it regularly, it will cease to function long before its expected life.

The most familiar example of mal-adaptation in the body is osteoarthrosis, aka degenerative arthritis. When bone is exposed to small forces over a prolonged period, it remodels itself (structural adaptation).

However, when bone undergoes too much structural adaptation, its new shape is no longer functional. Like rust on a bicycle chain, it interferes with movement, creates inflammation, and causes joint pain.

Once structural mal-adaptation occurs inside the body it is an irreversible process, which creates new problems in addition to the original one.

In short, mal-adaptation occurs when a temporary solution is not so temporary and thus becomes part of the greater problem.

CHAPTER 14

It's Complicated

*Do not forget that chiropractors did not treat dis-
eases. They adjust causes, whether acquired,
spontaneous, or the result of accident.*

DD Palmer

When muscle memory and structural mal-adaptation unite, they create the perfect storm for disaster in the upper cervical spine.

Step by step, here is what happens.

If your atlas has been misaligned for a long time, the continuous positional feedback from the sensors in your neck will convince your brain that this position is actually normal. Therefore your brain will tell your muscles to adopt new motor patterns, which effectively keep your atlas in this abnormal position.

The atlas subluxation is now resistant to change.

In order to maintain the balance of your head, your neck curve will decrease. This change exerts great stress on the joints of your lower neck. At the same time, your back curve will decrease, the result of which will be increased pressure on the discs of your lower back.

Like a contagious disease, this body imbalance problem spreads to all the joints in your body including your upper back, shoulders, hips and knees. The problem gets worse from there. After all your joints have been misaligned long enough, the continuous positional feedback will convince your brain that all these positions are normal.

As the saying goes, "If you repeat a lie often enough, it becomes the truth."

This corrupted feedback mechanism and the resultant muscle memory problem is the reason so many people's posture is not straight even though they feel that it is. Therefore your brain will tell your muscles to adopt abnormal motor patterns, which effectively lock your joints in improper positions.

Your entire body is now resistant to change.

To accommodate the elevated amounts of stress, muscles and ligaments throughout your body reshape: that is, they undergo structural adaptation.

"If your head is not on straight, it wants to plop down," explains Dr Tom Forest. "[Because] we need to keep the head level for equilibrium and balance reasons, the muscles from the base of the skull to the bottom of the neck—the upper thoracic area—have to tighten and shorten to keep the head upright. So you end up having atrophy, dried up muscles on the anterior [front of the neck], and hypertrophy or thickened muscles on the posterior [back of the neck].

"This is frequently why people need to have their shoulders rubbed all the time because those muscles are just so tight and rigid. The irony is if you have this rigidity, you can go to Hawaii and relax as much as you want, but the muscles are just as rigid as can be because they're mechanically having to hold that head up."
cxlviii

Strong tissues will get stronger, shorter, thicker and tighter. Weak tissues will get weaker, longer, thinner and more flaccid.

That is the evolutionary process that turns a relatively simple upper cervical problem into such a complex and resilient monster.

Remember that physical trauma is what causes an upper cervical subluxation in the first place. Usually it is something significant like a direct blow to the head or a repetitive stress injury. If that injury is not corrected and left untouched for weeks, months or years, then it may only take a small amount of stress to disrupt the balance.

On the surface, everything may appear calm. However, like a dormant volcano the problem will become abundantly apparent should that volcano erupt!

Much like the straw that breaks the camel's back, there is only so much physical adaptation and stress that your body can handle before it snaps. More often than not, that straw is just an innocent activity like getting out of bed, reversing your car from the driveway, sweeping the floor, sitting in the car or doing computer work.

It is strange that many people do not associate their current state of health with events that happened long ago. Nevertheless, it is only when an innocent activity triggers pain that many people finally learn the full extent of their hidden problems

---

Case Report: Emily's Story (Part II)

> I wanted to know what had caused Emily's problems in the first place.
>
> "Has she had memorable injuries? Falls, bumps or hits to the head? Anything like that?"
>
> "Ugh ..." Christine groaned, shaking her head.

"Well," Emily started grinning with delight, "There was the time I fell off the ladder from the roof. And we have a trampoline, so I've fallen off that a few times too. That was fun. And last year I got hit in the head with the football playing Oz Tag. I got tackled a bunch of times too."

"I thought Oz Tag was a non-contact sport?" I enquired.

"Not when our teacher makes us play. He loves Oz Tag. We have to play almost every day. The boys always try to tackle the girls, and they're really rough about it."

"She was black and blue all the way up her side for a week last year," Christine added.

"I hate Oz Tag," Emily finished emphatically.

"What about when you fell off the horse?" Christine asked Emily.

"Oh yeah," Emily started again. "I fell off a horse when I was five. And I've fallen down the stairs a couple of times too."

Emily could not stop smiling as she recounted the numerous major injuries she had suffered in her short life. It was as if each incident was a badge of honour.

Christine and Emily carried on like this for another 10 minutes. When they could no longer recall any other injuries, I recommended that I examine her to see if there was any way that I could help her.

"Is it going to hurt?" Emily asked with a hint of fear in her voice.

"It's not going to hurt," I responded. "I promise."

Just like all her specialists before me, I found nothing bizarre during her exam. On the positive side, it meant that Emily did not have any exotic disease, tumour or infection. On the other hand, it meant that something else was causing her condition.

I next performed an Upper Cervical examination for Emily. It was quite the challenge! Her body was so twisted that she was unable to lie flat on the examination table.

Nevertheless, I was able to measure her leg length inequality: well over 15cm shorter on the left side. I could also feel a tremendous amount of tension through her upper neck and sacrum (lower back around the tailbone).

I was certain that Emily had a subluxation, which was likely caused by one of her many injuries. I also had a theory as to why Emily's body was rebelling against her so fiercely.

The spinal cord tethers onto the vertebral column at only two sites: the atlas and the sacrum. With both of these areas significantly misaligned, I imagined that Emily's spinal cord had been strapped inside a proverbial torture rack and was getting stretched to its breaking point. I believed that the resulting tension was creating so much neural interference that it was causing her body to spasm and contort.

I proceeded to explain my theory to Christine and Emily. I also explained to them the nature of Upper Cervical care: to unlock the vertebrae, to take the pressure off her nervous system, to clear her body of neural interference and then allow her body to heal on its own.

Given the severe natures of Emily's presentation, I did not believe Upper Cervical care alone would be the complete solution for her. She also needed significant work to unlock her lower back.

At Palmer, I had studied sacro-occipital therapy (SOT) under Dr Vern Hagen, who in his younger years was one of the leaders for SOT in the world. In his later years, Dr Hagen would also become one of the greatest allies for Upper Cervical care.

"There is no conflict," I remember Dr Hagen saying. "SOT and Upper Cervical complement each other: the atlas at the top and the sacrum at the bottom of the spine."

Honestly, I had no idea if this combination of Upper Cervical and SOT would be able to help, but as I explained to Christine and Emily, the only way we would ever know would be to try.

(Continued in Chapter 20)

Three Causes

Even before the discovery of neurotransmitters, muscle memory and structural mal-adaptation, the founder of chiropractic, DD Palmer, identified three things that disrupt normal nerve function:
- physical injuries,
- chemical sensitivities, and
- thoughts and emotions.

With any complex upper cervical problem, any small amount of these stimuli may be enough to aggravate a nerve and trigger symptoms.

First, let us consider physical injuries.

A simple trauma such as bumping your head on a car door or kitchen cupboard may be enough to aggravate a chronic subluxation. Micro-trauma like sleeping on a couch or in a foreign bed may be sufficient to trigger symptoms. Even doing simple repetitive activities like washing your hair, working on a computer or playing golf may be enough to spark an injury.

That is one of the most unfortunate consequences of a chronic subluxation: it may not take any major force at all to cause injury or pain!

Second, let's consider chemical sensitivities. Imagine that you are refueling your car at a petrol station. You may not have a sensitivity to gasoline fumes, but if you were to stand there for a full day, you would likely have a few mild symptoms of chemical poisoning (e.g., headache).

Now imagine that you also have an upper cervical subluxation. All it may take now is for you to stand around petrol fumes for a few minutes before you suffer a headache. The presence of a chronic subluxation lowers the threshold necessary for internal and external chemicals to disrupt normal human physiology.

A chemical overload may trigger a huge range of problems from headaches, nausea and lightheadness to skin rashes, indigestion or diarrhea. Just as there are an infinite number of physical triggers, so too are there countless chemical triggers.

A few examples things that people ingest would include alcohol, caffeine, chocolate, gluten or dairy—not failing to mention the food additives, preservatives, hormones and pesticides that are present in many food-like products.

Chemical stimuli may also include things that you inhale deliberately or accidentally from the environment such as cigarette smoke, industrial fumes, dust, pollen or mold. You may even have a sensitivity to something you put into your hair or skin: dyes, perfumes, lotions, sunscreens, and all the synthetic chemicals that are used to manufacture them.

———

Finally, let's examine thoughts and emotional disturbances.

For simplicity, these types of triggers may be summarized in one word: stress. As I have said before, we cannot disconnect our thoughts and emotions from our bodies.

As far as the nervous system is concerned, mental impulses are the same as physical impulses. They just use a different combination of neurotransmitters to convey a slightly different message.

Any radical shift in thought has the potential to disrupt your wellbeing. Events like a flat tire, a broken-down vehicle, an unexpected bill or the death of a loved one may trigger stress.

One of the major problems with people in today's world is chronic stress. Living with an abusive spouse, dealing with whining kids, working in an unpleasant environment, running a business, paying the mortgage, caring for an elderly parent: the list goes on and on!

Chronic stress may contribute to a number of psychological disorders including anxiety, depression, post-traumatic stress syndrome, or any other disorder that creates a vicious disease cycle within the body and mind.

To complicate matters, not only is your nervous system affected by chronic stress, so are your endocrine (hormone) and immune systems. Any shift of these systems from the normal also has the potential to trigger symptoms. Hormone cycles (male and female), pregnancy, infections (bacterial, viral or fungal including candida) and other disease states such as cancer all have the potential to create physiological stress and trigger symptoms within the body.

The list I have just described is far from all-inclusive. It is only the tip of the iceberg. However, I believe it should be clear just how many things could affect a subluxation if it becomes chronic.

Truly, it is a complex problem!

———————————————

Nerve sensors translate all types of stimuli—physical, chemical and emotional—into the same language (neurotransmitters) for the brain to interpret and act upon.

That is the reason so many different stimuli all have the same effect on your body.

That is also the reason so many different stimuli cause chronic upper cervical problems to relapse and trigger a new wave of pain and dysfunction.

As I have mentioned previously, people often assume that if they suffer an injury but walk away without any blood or broken bones that they must be healthy. This assumption is not always true.

Unfortunately it is the exact reason that so many people have complex upper cervical spinal problems.

If a person seeks Upper Cervical treatment at the time of the original trauma, the problem usually resolves quickly and easily. To use an analogy, it is easier to stop the momentum of a rolling snowball at the top of a mountain than at the bottom. Alas, many people do not seek Upper Cervical care until they are buried beneath an avalanche of health problems.

That is why an atlas problem—a relatively simple problem—can become so complex and resistant to correction.

CHAPTER 15

Beneath the Surface

When you see, you know. When you don't see, you guess.

Dr BJ Palmer

Since its incorporation into the Palmer School in 1909, x-ray has played an integral part for the advancement of Upper Cervical care. Computed axial tomography (CT or CAT scans), magnetic resonance imaging (MRI) and other advanced studies have greatly assisted medical science over the past decades.

It is unfortunate that these modalities have not lent themselves as viable, cost-effective options for chiropractic use. X-ray remains the gold standard diagnostic procedure for Upper Cervical chiropractic practice.

Most Upper Cervical doctors require at least three views are required to see the atlas and axis in three-dimensions:
- a side or lateral view (Figure 15.1);
- a horizontal view, aka Base-Posterior or Vertex (Figure 15.2); and
- a frontal view, aka Nasium (Figure 15.3).

Many Upper Cervical doctors also take oblique nasium or protracto views (Figure 15.4 and Figure 15.5) in order to clearly see the exact location and degree of atlas misalignment. As stated by Dr William Blair, the developer of this x-ray view, "If the misalignment happens at the joint, why not take a picture of the joint to see the misalignment?"

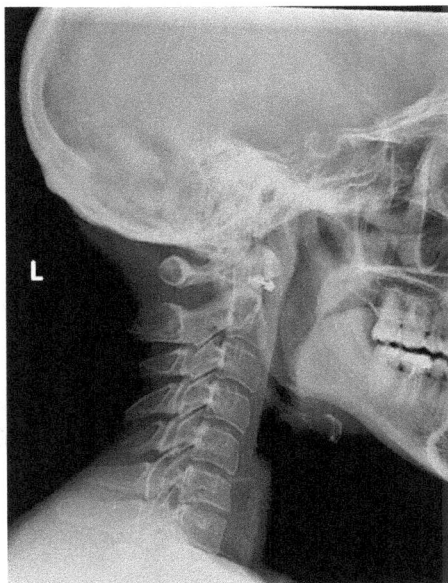

Figure 15.1 Lateral X-Ray.

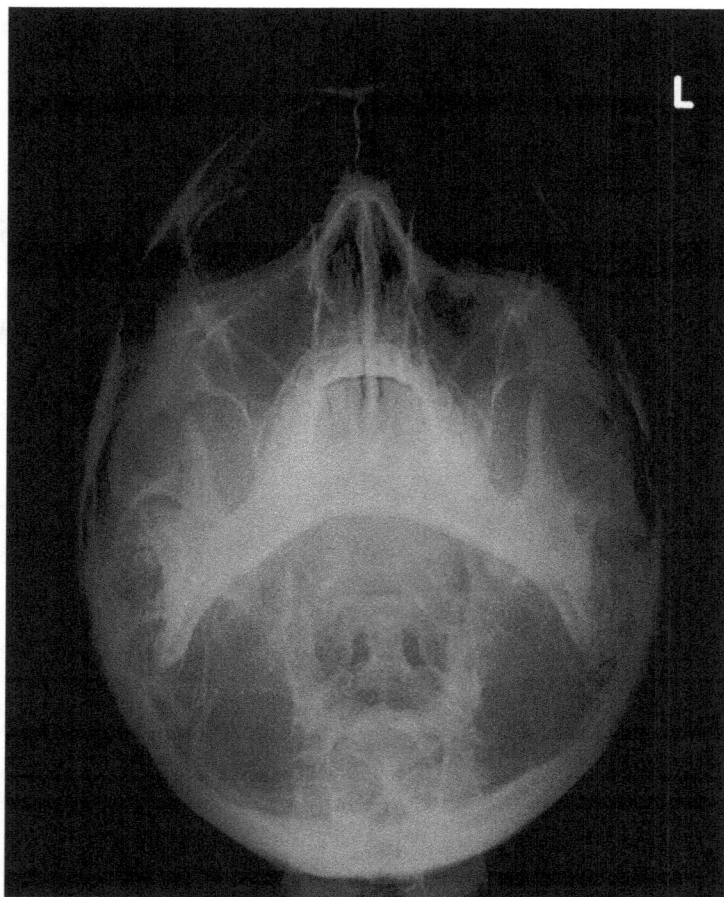

Figure 15.2 Horizontal X-Ray.

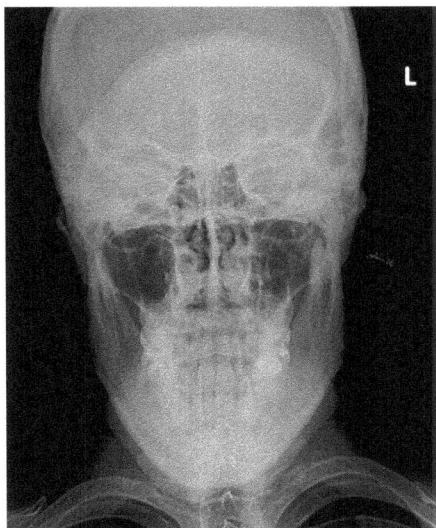

Figure 15.3 Frontal X-Ray.

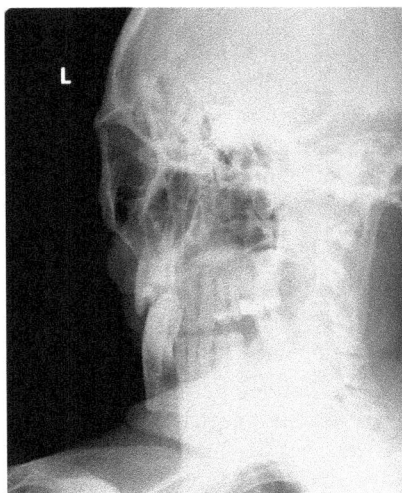

Figure 15.4 Left Protracto X-Ray.

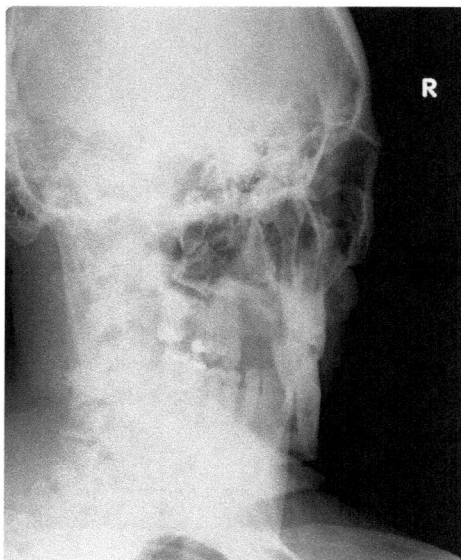

15.5 Right Protracto X-Ray.

It is also standard protocol to take two sets of x-rays: a pre series that shows the misalignment; and a post series that shows improvement after the correction.

Having a before-and-after comparison is essential for an Upper Cervical chiropractor to gauge the effectiveness of the treatment and to see if there is any fine-tuning that is still needed.

Numerous studies have demonstrated strong reliability and validity of Upper Cervical x-ray analysis. [cxlix cl cli clii] One study in particular demonstrated that patients experience better outcomes if the total misalignment is reduced by at least 50% as determined by x-rays. [cliii]

One major difference between standard x-rays and Upper Cervical precision x-rays is the meticulous attention to detail that doctors take to ensure that the images show a true biomechanical picture of the upper neck.

All precision x-rays are taken in a neutral position: that is, the posture that you believe is straight and upright. Remember the phenomenon of body imbalance? Look again at old pictures of yourself, or look in a mirror. Is your head on straight?

If not, this is the problem that Upper Cervical chiropractors aim to measure. If your head naturally leans forward, your doctor will want to see that on x-ray. Or if your head tilts or turns to one side, your doctor will want to see that as well.

If a radiographer changes the neutral position of your head so that it is centred for the picture, it nullifies the reason for taking the x-ray in the first place.

The neutral position is where an Upper Cervical chiropractor measures the amount of atlas misalignment and determines the best way to fix the problem.

Interestingly, there is no correlation between the intensity of a person's symptoms and the magnitude of an upper cervical misalignment. Some people have huge atlas displacements but relatively minor symptoms. Other people have tiny misalignments but massive health problems. I have seen this phenomenon in my own practice, and it has been reported by many other Upper Cervical chiropractors as well. [cliv clv]

However, there does appear to be a connection between symptom intensity and the pattern of misalignment: i.e., into the kink and counter-rotational patterns.

Lateral tilting patterns (Figure 15.6 and Figure 15.7) involve the relative amount of head tilt with respect to the lower neck. That is, do the head and neck tilt in opposing directions (e.g., the head to the right and the neck to the left), or do they tilt toward the same side?

The latter pattern is known as an into the kink pattern and is often regarded as the more problematic of the two. It is hypothesized that the dentate ligaments exert greater physiological stress on the spinal cord when an into the kink pattern is present. Greater tension tends to cause problems associated with the spinocerebellar tracts: body imbalance, associated musculoskeletal injuries and associated pain syndromes. [clvi clvii]

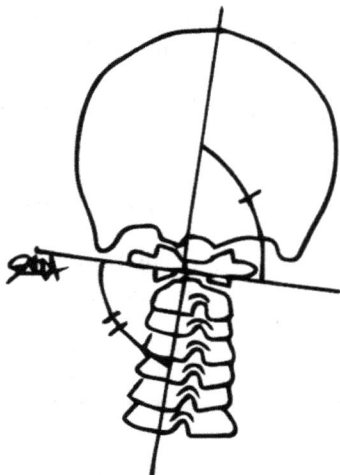

Figure 15.6 Normal Compensation Tilting Pattern.

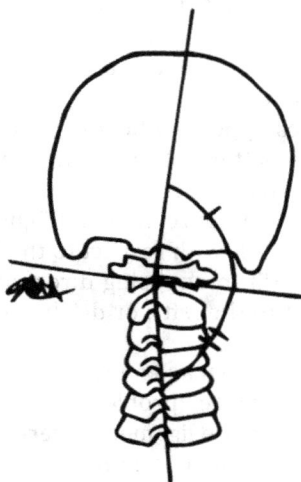

Figure 15.7 Into the Kink Tilting Pattern.

Rotational patterns (Figure 15.8) involve the relative amount of C1 twisting respect to C2. That is, do they both rotate toward the same side or do they rotate in opposite directions?

When the top two vertebrae rotate in opposite directions (i.e., counter-rotate) they cause torsional stress on the spinal cord. It is much the same as if you are wringing out a dishcloth. This type of stress tends to produce symptoms associated with the corticospinal and the spinothalamic tracts: motor problems, balance disruptions and neurologic pain syndromes (e.g., trigeminal neuralgia). [clviii]

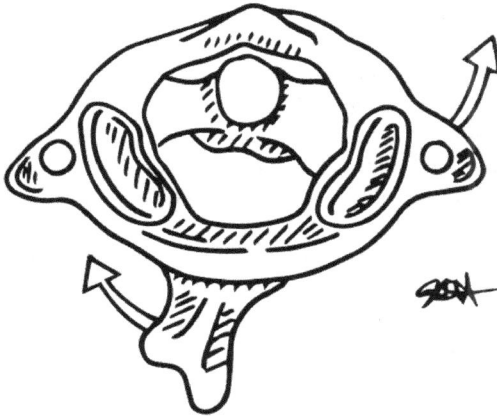

Figure 15.8 Counter-rotational Patterns.

Case Report: Trigeminal Neuralgia

Tony was a 50 year-old gentle giant of a man, who was referred by his orthodontist.

"Doc calls it trigeminal neuralgia."

Tony spoke eloquently but with a few peculiarities: he always used short sentences, and he seldom used subject pronouns like "I" or "He." He also had an audible clicking noise coming from his jaw.

"It started when I had a tooth extraction four years ago. Dentist said I needed the tooth out. He lay me back in his chair. Gave me the anaesthetic. That was it. That night I feel this jolt in me jaw. Didn't think much of it. Two weeks later, it's still happening.

"Went to see the specialists. Did scans of me jaw and head. Everything's fine, so they just gave me these tablets. Tablets didn't do a thing, so they gave me more. Still didn't do a thing. I don't like tablets anyway, so I just gave them up.

"Last year I decided to see this dentist, who says he can help. Doc tells me I have arthritis in me jaw, which is the reason it clicks. Tells me it's not going to go away.

"Also says my jaw is crooked, but he can fix that. Six months later, he's done wonders! I've got a splint, which has let me chew again. I've stopped grinding me teeth. And me jaw is much straighter.

"But I'm still getting the pain when I have tea in the evenings. Last week Doc does a few more tests. Tells me he thinks it's my neck and says I should see you.

"Most of the time its okay. But its only when I'm having me tea at night.

"When it grabs," he winced with a grimace on his face, "it's like lightning. But if I move my neck it eventually stops."

As part of my examination, I checked all of Tony's cranial nerves. Although I did not detect any abnormalities with his trigeminal nerve, I did note some significant problems with the nerve that controls the muscles of facial expression (see Bell's palsy in Chapter 4).

"I was in me 20s when I got jumped in a bar," Tony recalled. "Two fellows started causing trouble with this young lady. I stepped in trying to help her. Some fellow hits me from behind with a bottle. That's all I remember.

"I wake up in the hospital the next day with me mouth wired shut. Docs tell me I broke me jaw, cheek and eye socket. Also said I damaged me facial nerve. Didn't know if it'd come back, but it's gotten a lot better since then."

Looking at Tony's x-rays, his atlas was definitely misaligned. Although the total amount of misalignment was relatively small, his atlas and axis were counter-rotated, which did correlate with the types of symptoms he was experiencing.

Tony also had a considerable amount of arthritic damage through his neck. Although I could not prove it, I believed it was very likely that Tony's assault 30 years ago was the actual cause of his problems. His visit to the dentist was probably just the catalyst that triggered his symptoms.

I adjusted Tony and recommended that I see him again in a couple of days.

"I'm on call for work for the next fortnight, so I'll call you when
I'm able to come."

I respected Tony's wishes and waited for him to contact me. When he contacted me two weeks later, he had nothing but positive news to report.

"No pain. Sorry I forgot to call earlier. Just slipped me mind. But no pain at all. Thought it was going to play up that first night, but I did me neck stretches and it never came.

"I didn't think it'd do anything," Tony added referring to his treatment, "but that the first full week in four years everything's felt normal."

Tony was not yet out of the woods, but for him to experience such significant relief after only one treatment was a definite step in the right direction. The good news kept coming when I checked Tony's neck the following day.

"Your adjustment is holding in place. I'm not going to do anything."

Because Tony's work schedule prohibited a proper check up, I instructed him to give a call if the problem came back even once.

A week passed, and I did not hear from Tony. Then another week. Then a month. I did not actually hear from Tony again until three months after his first treatment.

"Still no pain. Neck feeling real good. Just wanted to let you know."

It was the best news that Tony could have shared.

I explain to people that the perfect Upper Cervical correction is the one that I perform only once and holds forever. Many people do experience significant relief with their first Upper Cervical treatment. However, the notion that just one treatment will permanently cure anyone is usually not true. The reasons will be explained in later chapters.

Although most people do not experience such complete and long-lasting relief with just a single adjustment, Tony's case does illustrate that it does happen. When it does—when the pain that people have suffered for so long disappears like it was never there—it is always a wonderful occasion.

As an important closing comment for anyone suffering trigeminal neuralgia, I strongly recommend that you read the amazing story of Mr James Tomasi in his book *What TIME Tuesday?*

Mr Tomasi's story of suffering for 15 years before discovering Upper Cervical care, a discovery that literally saved his life is one of the most compelling and inspirational stories I have ever read. Mr Tomasi and his wife Rhonda have since become two of the strongest advocates for Upper Cervical care in the world.

For more information and to read *What TIME Tuesday?* visit their website:
www.uppercervicaladvocates.com.

Medical radiologists use x-rays to look for problems such as fractures, dislocations, arthritis and certain diseases. General chiropractors go one step further to see the biomechanical relationships of the spinal vertebrae. In other words, they look for relative amounts of misalignment: e.g., the axis is misaligned in a posterior, right and inferior direction (PRI).

Upper Cervical chiropractors go one step farther to determine the exact amount of misalignment: e.g., the atlas is misaligned 20 degrees to the right and 5 degrees posterior, and the axis is counter-rotated 10 degrees to the left.

Dr Susan Brown describes it another way. "If you ask [people] directions to some place, and they say 'Head down here and turn left at the tree,' it's the difference between that and going to MapQuest where you have exactly the right information on how to get there."

She adds, "The information that we give as Upper Cervical doctors to the body to allow it to heal is so much more specific and so much more precise ... that the body is able to take that information and run with it. So people get well quickly and stay well." [clix]

CHAPTER 16

Don't Play Guessing Games

All truth goes through three stages. First, it is ridiculed. Second, it is violently opposed. Third, it is accepted as being self-evident.

Arthur Schopenhauer

Many people ask the question, "Do I need to have x-rays?"

Would you ever drive a car with your eyes closed? Would you ever play darts in the dark? Or would you ever ask a surgeon to work on you while wearing a blindfold?

Of course not! It boils down to one simple thing: risk.

So why people believe that it is okay to seek upper cervical treatment without x-rays absolutely baffles me. For an Upper Cervical chiropractor (or anyone else for that matter) to work without an x-ray is unwise, unsafe and extremely unlikely to get you the results you're seeking.

Dr Kirk Eriksen is one of the world leaders in Upper Cervical practice and research. Among his numerous contributions is a particular study, where he examined if an upper cervical misalignment could be predicted accurately with any non-radiographic method.

Dr Eriksen considered a number of methods including kinesiology, thermography (the study of temperature differentials), posture analysis, and static and motion palpation where the chiropractor feels through the skin to determine the relative direction of misalignment.

His results were quite remarkable. Not a single one of these non-radiographic methods consistently predicted the true position of the atlas or axis, which appeared on the x-ray as plain as day. [clx]

Dr Eriksen concluded, "While non-radiographic methods might be useful as pre- and post-adjustment screening checks, they should not be relied on to provide misalignment listings for adjustment." [clxi]

He would add later, "Radiographic analysis is the closest thing to a 'gold' standard for assessing the biomechanics of the upper cervical spine." [clxii]

Precise measurement is a critical factor when considering an atlas misalignment. Few would argue that one degree is structurally important for a mechanical engineer or that a single millimetre is functionally important for a neurosurgeon.

So too are such small measurements vitally important for an Upper Cervical chiropractor.

Scientists estimate that there are 1,000,000 neurons in one cubic millimetre (mm^3) of the brainstem. [clxiii] If one degree of misalignment creates neurological tension or disrupts blood flow to just 1.0 mm^3 of brain tissue, the health consequences could be enormous.

Read the first section of this book again if you doubt that statement!

If one degree of misalignment may cause so many problems, so too may one degree of correction be the key to restoring health.

It is the reason that Upper Cervical chiropractors undergo the extensive training that they do. When such a tiny difference can affect so many things in the body, it behooves anyone who works in the upper neck region to approach it with the same level of respect, precision and care as a neurosurgeon.

To reiterate the words of BJ Palmer, "Chiropractic is specific or it is nothing."

To add to this statement, I would like to add that it is far better to be more specific than necessary than not specific enough.

Only with precision x-rays are Upper Cervical doctors able to determine the degree of vertebral misalignment with confidence.

Safety

I believe that most objections about x-rays involve some aspect of personal safety.

Let us first consider the amount of radiation actually used in an Upper Cervical x-ray examination.

The average person in Australia or the United States is exposed to 2 milliSieverts (mSv) of radiation per year from natural background sources including the sun and the environment. [clxiv] By comparison, compare the amount of x-ray exposure for the following common diagnostic procedures:

- lumbar x-ray   1.5 mSv;
- head CT scan   2.0 mSv;
- spinal CT scan   6.0 mSv; and
- chest CT scan   7.0 mSv. [clxv]

The radiation from an Upper Cervical x-ray series, which includes pre- and post- views, is only 0.15-0.30 mSv. [clxvi]

This dosage is comparable to a few weeks of natural radiation or to 15-hour flight from Australia to the United States. [clxvii] Radiation experts estimate that the chance of developing cancer from such a minimal level of radiation is only one per 100,000 – 1,000,000 individuals. [clxviii]

On the other end of the spectrum, consider that the amount of radiation used in cancer treatment varies between 20,000 to 80,000 mSv depending on the aggressiveness of the disease. [clxix]

I hope that these numbers illustrate that there is a major difference between the large amount of radiation that may cause acute illness and the relatively small amount of radiation used for diagnostic imaging.

The International Commission of Radiological Protection (ICRP) has recommended that the public should not be exposed routinely to more than 1.0 mSv above natural levels in one year, but that health professionals should not be exposed to more than 20.0 mSv. [clxx]

Thus, on the concern that x-ray exposure may cause cancer, it is not the person who is exposed to one x-ray who is at risk: it is the radiographer who takes multiple exposures each and every day.

Overall, the risk of suffering health complications from a single Upper Cervical x-ray is minimal at best.

━━━━━━━━━━

A second point to consider is the clinical benefit of having an x-ray.

Consider the example of a cancer patient. Despite the consequences of radiation therapy (e.g., hair loss, skin lesions and weakness), those problems may be better than the alternate option—death.

Another example would be a pregnant woman, who is involved in a serious car accident. If there is the possibility that she has broken her neck, the risk of that injury greatly outweighs the risk of radiation exposure to her unborn child. Thus, an x-ray may be necessary to save them both.

There is a simple but vital code of ethics that all professionals, who work with ionizing radiation must uphold:

When the risk of x-ray exposure if greater than the risk of not taking the x-ray, do not take the x-ray. Conversely, when the risk of not doing the x-ray is greater than taking it, the procedure is justified.

Upper Cervical chiropractors consider several factors before recommending x-rays including the patient's age, the severity of their condition, and the degree to which it is affecting their quality of life. Personally, I do not recommend Upper Cervical x-rays for children under 8 years unless they are suffering severe neurological problems. I also do not recommend x-rays for pregnant women, who can usually wait for x-rays until after they have given birth.

When a person truly desires a solution for their health issues, precision x-ray is the best and only way to see with absolute certainty how to correct the problem. When even one millimetre may be significant, to treat the problem without x-ray is not advised and may even be dangerous.

Congenital Anomalies

A congenital anomaly refers to any different way that your bones develop when you were born or growing up. A few common examples include things such as a cervical rib (an extra nub of bone that extends from the lower part of the neck), a hip dysplasia or a hammertoe.

Congenital anomalies are usually not anything dangerous or scary, but it does mean that a person's biomechanics are not the same as everyone else.

Dr William Blair, founder of the Blair method deserves great credit for his extensive work with anatomical variations and for developing ways to accommodate them when correcting upper cervical subluxations.

I have seen cases where the atlas is fused with the head, where it is fused with the axis, and where the back portion of both C1 and C2 are missing entirely. I have seen other cases where the atlas had been fractured and healed. I have even seen one case where the atlas was still split in two separate pieces. [clxxi]

The short of it, most congenital anomalies cannot be palpated through the skin and can only be detected with an x-ray. It is yet another important reason for Upper Cervical doctors to see what is going on with the neck before they attempt to treat it.

————————

I don't play guessing games with my own health. Likewise, I do not play games with the health of my patients.

Let me tell a story to illustrate the point. Imagine that y

One day you start to experience some uncomfortable symptoms. You go to see a general chiropractor who does not take an x-ray. If the chiropractor goes by palpation alone to feel the more-prominent bony landmark, he may assume that your atlas is misaligned toward the left side.

He adjusts you and you get worse! What happened?

You decide to see another chiropractor who does take an x-ray. Guess what he finds? It turns out that you have a congenital anomaly. The transverse process (bony protrusion on the left side of your atlas) is larger than the one on the right side.

So even though it may feel like the atlas needs to be adjusted from the left side, the exact opposite is true. The atlas is actually misaligned toward the right side.

No wonder your symptoms got worse after your first "adjustment!"

Although this may sound like a rare occurrence, it is not. I feel it very important to caution you not to allow any health practitioner to work on your neck without first taking an x-ray.

I learnt this lesson long ago, for it was this very error that caused Joe's problems in the first place.

Yes, the same "Joe" you've been reading about throughout this book. Go back to Chapter 3 and re-read what Kevin told me had happened right before Joe's symptoms started: "He was at the student clinic last Friday, and they were working on his neck."

For all the hurried frenzy that was happening that morning, Dr Hannah and I still took the time to review Joe's file. Sure enough, we discovered that he did have his atlas manipulated on the left side.

As a preview of what we were about to discover, we would learn two important things from Joe's x-rays that his other intern did not know: he had an enlarged atlas transverse process on the left side ... but his atlas was misaligned toward the right side.

That is the importance of seeing.

When you see you know. When you don't see, you guess.

Part III

Art

Interlude II

To know and not to do, is to not know at all.

Bruce Lee

Beep.
Beep.
Beep.

The first three x-rays were the routine cervical spine series. The measurements that we would take from these pictures would allow us to calculate the angles needed to take the next two Upper Cervical x-rays.

I slipped out of the room to check with Dr Hannah and Louise, who were examining the images on the computer screen.

"Nothing out of the ordinary except for the curve of his neck," my dad commented. Sure enough, Joe's neck, which should have been curved forward, was curved in the opposite direction.

After measuring the alignment of the atlas, I returned to Joe. I didn't know how much longer he could tolerate sitting upright with the lights in his eyes. Without any margin for error, I knew that the next two x-rays had to be perfect.

I opted to take the frontal view first because it would be the easiest to setup. Plus Joe was already sitting in the correct position. I checked that he maintained his head in what he believed was his neutral position. I also made sure his head was stabilized and aligned centrally with the x-ray beam.

Everything looked good.

Beep.

The last x-ray was the horizontal view, which I expected would be hardest for Joe because it would require him to lean forward so that his chin could rest on the flat surface of the x-ray board.

As I helped Joe into position, I was quite surprised when he commented that this setup was actually the most comfortable of the lot. I made certain that his face was not rotated and that his chin was aligned with the centre of the film. With his head stabilized, we took the last x-ray.

Beep.

"That's it, Joe."

Kevin was quick to attend to Joe, whom I'm certain was completely exhausted by now. Again I popped out of the room to check with my dad.

"What do you think?" he asked as the image appeared on the screen.

Without as much practice as my dad, it took me a little longer to figure out what I was seeing.

"He looks like his head is tilting to the right," I responded, "but his C2 is rotating backwards to the left."

"It also looks like his left transverse process is enlarged," he added. "Its pretty close when you look at it, but based on the slope of the condyles [the smooth elliptical surfaces of the skull that articulate with the atlas], he should be adjusted from the right side."

He then added, "Can you do the analysis?"

As much as I had wanted a lazy day just an hour earlier, I couldn't think of anywhere more important to be.

"I'll have it in 15 minutes."

I once heard the story of a young man, who trained for many years to earn a black belt in karate. Upon completing his examination, he presented before his Sensei (teacher) who asked him one question: "What does the black belt mean to you?"

Eagerly, the young man responded, "The black belt is the ending of my journey. It is the reward for my years of hard work."

The Sensei bowed softly to the young man but replied, "I am sorry. You are not ready. You may try again next year."

The young man could not believe this reversal of fortune. He was consumed by anger for many days. Eventually he chose to focus harder on his training. One year later, he returned for the examination. Again, his Sensei asked him, "What does the black belt mean to you?"

Confidently, the man responded, "The black belt is the ending of my journey. It symbolizes patience and persistence."

Again, the Sensei bowed but responded the same way. "I am sorry. You are not ready. You may try again next year."

The man was beside himself. Again he was consumed by rage, but this time for many weeks. However, he again chose to focus harder on his training. This time, he also focused inward to comprehend why his Sensei had twice denied him his prize.

One year later, he returned for the examination. A third time, his Sensei asked, "What does the black belt mean to you?

Wisely and with humility, the man responded, "The black belt is not the ending of my journey. It is the beginning."

The Sensei then said with a smile, "Yes, now you are ready." He then bowed to the man and presented him with his black belt.

I will admit freely that I am still an Upper Cervical student. Although I have practiced for several years now, I have a long way to go before truly mastering the art.

In the first section of this book, we discussed the reasons that an upper cervical misalignment can cause such a wide variety of health problems. In the second section, we've examined the simple and complex causes of the subluxation.

In the final section of this book, we will look at Upper Cervical treatment, how it differs from general chiropractic, but also how it works alongside other forms of healthcare.

Before we proceed, I would like to make a strange but important comment: don't believe anything that I have written in this book thus far.

That's right. I want you to completely ignore everything that you've just read.

As a doctor, I have seen how Upper Cervical care changes lives. Unless you are also a doctor, you may not have had the same opportunity. For all the stories I've detailed in this book, if I had not seen many of these transformations with my own eyes, I would probably still have my own doubts.

Therefore, it is important that you not simply take my word for it, but that you do your own research and then make up your own mind.

One of the most passionate advocates for Upper Cervical care, whom I have had the fortune to meet is, Mr Greg Buchanan. Greg has a voracious appetite for knowledge, and since his life-changing experience with Upper Cervical care has extensively studied all the evidence, validity and science behind it.

I should like to emphasize that Greg has no formal medical or chiropractic qualifications, but his knowledge on the subject is just as great as any Upper Cervical chiropractor I know.

Greg's story is so inspirational that it would never do him justice if I tried to summarize it. His story written in his own words can be found on his website, www.upcspine.com

For patients and doctors alike, Greg has collected a huge volume of research articles, links and more stories written by real Upper Cervical patients. As he says on his home page, "I have developed this website primarily as an information website for people desperately searching for answers to their medical conditions."

In addition to his work on UpCSpine, Greg was also a co-executive producer for the 2007 documentary *The Power of Upper Cervical*. He remains a highly sought-after speaker for Upper Cervical conferences worldwide.

Like Greg, seek your own answers. Gain knowledge. Despite the adage that, "Knowledge is power," I would argue that it is actually the use of knowledge that is power.

CHAPTER 17

Atlas Specialist

How wonderful the opportunity, how great the responsibility.

Dr John F Grostic

Primum non nocere.

First, do no harm. As with all health professionals, Upper Cervical chiropractors adhere to a code of ethics. I have sworn above all else to never do anything that may jeopardize a person's health.

The second vital responsibility of Upper Cervical chiropractors is to respect the innate healing power within the human body. It is not the doctor who heals: only your own body has that power. Hence, my role as a doctor is simply to facilitate that healing process.

A third responsibility for an Upper Cervical chiropractor is to work in the best interest of the patient. My responsibility is to offer hope, but never to provide false hope or promise miracles. I am also mandated to provide only the precise amount of treatment that is required to help a person during the healing process—no more and no less.

When To Adjust

I cannot emphasize enough the importance of having x-rays before any person receives an Upper Cervical spinal treatment.

Although it seemed apparent that Joe's symptoms were linked with his chiropractic treatment the previous week, neither my dad nor I believed that was the original cause of his problem. The structural change that we saw on his x-rays—i.e., his reversed neck curve—was a strong indicator that Joe had a long-standing problem. We believed that it was simple chance that the manipulation had triggered his problem to become symptomatic.

Upper Cervical chiropractors perform many tests in order to determine when it is appropriate to adjust the atlas. It should be stressed that they never take x-rays until after they have performed those tests.

Pre- and post- precision x-rays are the definitive measure of an Upper Cervical problem. In order to achieve the safest and best clinical results, all patients must have precision x-rays taken prior to their first treatment.

However, people do not require x-rays before every treatment.

Upper Cervical chiropractors have long observed that people's x-ray patterns or listings are usually stable for decades at a time. [clxxii] [clxxiii] Basically when an atlas subluxation relapses, it usually returns to the same position as the original misalignment.

You do not need an x-ray every time you require Upper Cervical treatment.

145

Although Upper Cervical x-rays demonstrate how a doctor should adjust, they do not indicate when the doctor should perform the correction.

In order to determine when to adjust, Upper Cervical chiropractors may perform a variety of objective tests. Each doctor may use a slightly different protocol to determine when to adjust the atlas. However, there are three common assessment methods used in most Upper Cervical practices:

- Palpation,
- A supine or prone leg check; and
- Instrumentation.

Palpation is a simple test where an Upper Cervical chiropractor feels the back of the upper neck for muscle tension, swelling or tenderness of the C1 and C2 nerve roots (Figure 17.1). Some Upper Cervical chiropractors may also feel for joint restrictions that may limit how much you are able to move your head.

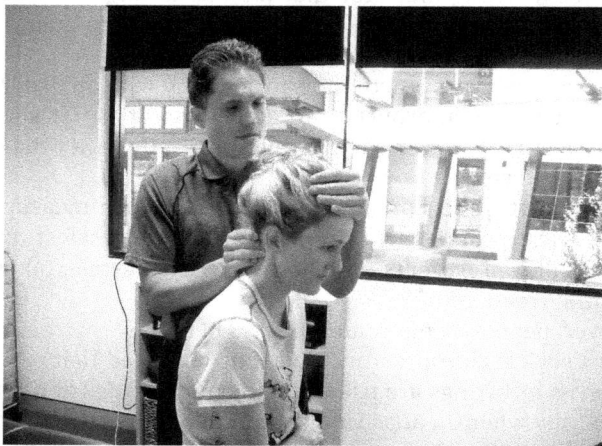

Figure 17.1. Palpation

A leg check is a test for body imbalance that can be performed with the patient lying either face-up (supine) or face-down (prone).

Remember that spinal cord tension creates asymmetrical muscle tension that remains whether you are standing, sitting or lying on a table (Figure 17.2).

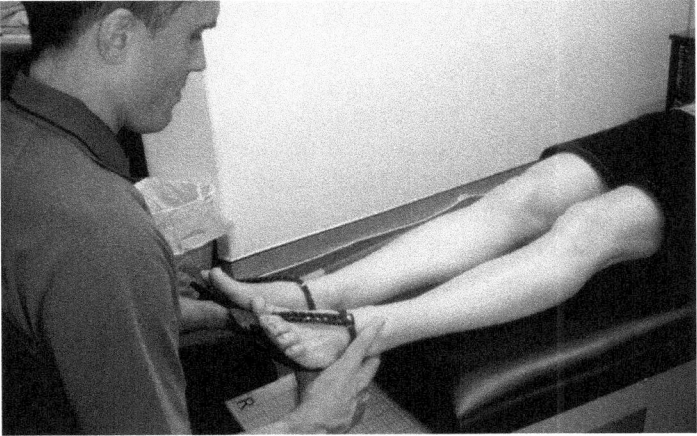

Figure 17.2. Leg Check (performed Supine).

Studies have shown that approximately 50% of the adult population has a short leg of 5 millimetres of more. If 5 mm sounds like an insignificant difference, I propose the following challenge: wear only one sock for a whole day. I think you will be (unpleasantly) surprised how sore your feet, knees, lower back and neck will feel.

Interestingly, Upper Cervical chiropractors find for approximately 90% of those people that the leg length inequality vanishes as soon as the atlas is adjusted. [clxxiv]

With the help of a spouse, friend or family member, you may be able to see for yourself if you have a leg length inequality.

- Wear a pair of hard-soled shoes and slide from the foot of your bed upward so that your ankles hang over the edge.

- Have your assistant stand over your feet with a camera and take a picture. If he or she cannot see much of a difference, repeat the process. The second time however, have your assistant apply equal pressure upward with his or her thumbs into the arches of both your shoes.

If one leg appears to be more than 5mm longer than the other, it is a reliable indicator of an atlas problem.

If you do the test supine (lying on your back), do so with a small pillow tucked under your head. If you do the test prone (lying on your stomach), you may want to see if there is any difference with the leg length inequality if you turn your head to the left or right. If so, that is an even stronger indicator for an upper cervical problem.

Not only do palpation and a supine/prone leg check provide valuable information if an Upper Cervical adjustment is required, they also provide immediate feedback on the effectiveness of the treatment. When a successful correction has been performed, both palpation and the body imbalance usually improve and within a few seconds.

―――――――――――

Instrumentation is the third type of test used to assess the upper neck. The most common instrumentation method is known as thermography, which is the study of temperature differentials along the spine (Figure 17.3).

Such practice actually dates back to ancient Greece. Hippocrates, the father of medicine would apply a thin layer of mud across a patient's back to observe where it dried fastest. An excerpt from Hippocrates' teachings reads that "Should one part of the body be hotter or colder than the rest, then disease is present in that part." clxxv

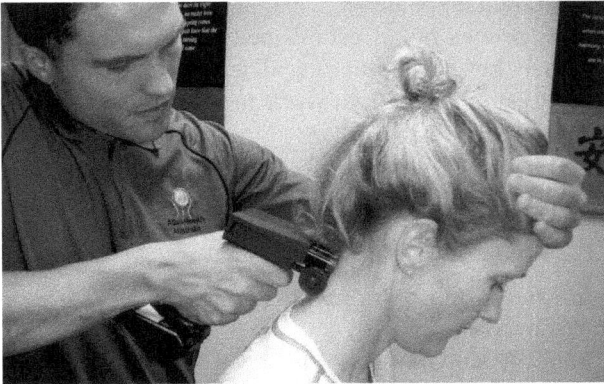

Figure 17.3. Thermography Scan.

The first instrument used for chiropractic purposes was the neurocalometer (NCM), which was introduced by BJ Palmer in 1924 amidst great acclaim and controversy.

As promoted by Dr Palmer, "The Neurocalometer is a very delicate, sensitive instrument which, when placed upon the spine:

- [It] verifies the proper places for adjustments.
- It measures the specific degree of vertebral pressures upon nerves.
- It measures the specific degree of interference to transmission of mental impulses as a result of vertebral pressure.
- It proves the exact intervertebral foramina that contains bone pressure upon nerves.

- It proves when the pressure has been released upon nerves at a specific place.
- It proves how much pressure was released, if any.
- It verifies the differences between cord pressure or spinal nerve pressure cases.
- It establishes which cases we can take and which we should leave alone.
- It proves by an established record, which you can see thereby eliminating all guess work on diagnoses.
- It establishes, from week to week, whether you are getting well or not.
- It makes possible a material reduction in time necessary to get well, thus making health cheaper." clxxvi

There are two primary forms of thermography: break analysis and pattern analysis.

Break analysis examines asymmetrical heat differentials on either side of the spine. A temperature difference as little as 0.30 degrees centigrade is a strong indicator that an upper cervical problem requires correction. A difference of 1.0 degree may even suggest the presence of outright disease such as an infection or tumor. clxxvii

Pattern analysis examines heat signatures along the spine. Each person has a unique temperature pattern that is like a fingerprint or ECG scan that shows when a person actually needs an atlas adjustment.

The NCM and other early thermography devices were thermocouples, instruments that measure temperature differentials when metal wires are placed on either sides of the spine. Modern thermography instruments now use laser scanners and even infrared cameras, which demonstrate temperature differences in vibrant colour.

Upper Cervical chiropractors may employ additional instrumentation methods to assess when to adjust. Such methods include computerized software that measures postural changes, surface electromyelographs (sEMGs) that measure regional muscle tension, and also digital scales that measure weight distribution.

You can perform this weight test for yourself using two simple bathroom scales. If you stand with your left foot on a scale and your right foot on a separate scale, your total body weight should be distributed evenly. When an atlas problem causes body imbalance, your body weight will not be distributed evenly.

Any leg length inequality greater than 6 millimetres usually shifts the excessive weight to the longer leg side. Inequality less than 6 mm usually shifts the weight to the shorter leg side. Irrespective, any weight differential beyond 3% (7 pounds, or 6% of your total body weight) indicates the need for an Upper Cervical correction. clxxviii clxxix

---

The tests that Upper Cervical doctors perform help to determine when an atlas correction is required. However, it is just as important for Upper Cervical chiropractors to know when to adjust as it is when not to adjust.

- When you do not have any palpable tension or pain in your neck;
- When you do not have a body imbalance problem;
- When your legs appear level;
- When instrument readings are within normal limits;
- But most important, when your body is functioning properly, you don't need an adjustment.

As Dr Drew Hall states, "What we want to see with patients is not to adjust them 5000 times over the life of their care. Our goal is to make a specific correction, unlock the vertebra, put it back in its

normal range of motion and keep it there for as long as possible."
clxxx

I often say to people, "If your adjustment isn't holding in place and if you have to keep coming back every couple of weeks, one of two things is happening. Number one, I've missed something, and I need to figure out what it is. Or number two, you're doing something that really isn't good for you, we need to figure out what it is, and then you need to figure out how you can change it."

Not needing an adjustment is a good thing. As the old saying goes, "If it ain't broke, don't fix it."

When your adjustment is holding, your body is healing.

CHAPTER 18

Risk versus Risky

Have you more faith in a knife or a spoonful of
medicine than in the power that
animates the living world?

Dr BJ Palmer

All things in life contain some element of risk: flying in an air-plane, swimming in the ocean, and even crossing a busy street. Upper Cervical treatment is no exception.

However, there is a big difference between risk and risky.

For example, driving a car has certain risks associated with it. If you drive defensively, wear your seatbelt and keep your focus on the road, you reduce your risk. On the other hand, if you have a few drinks, speed down the wrong side of the road and chat on your phone, you greatly increase your risk.

Upper Cervical care is a specialist practice with an unparalleled benefit-to-risk ratio, and an even better safety record associated with it.

However, this record only applies for Upper Cervical chiropractors and not other so-called atlas therapists, who seldom have the qualifications to treat disorders of the upper neck safely or effectively.

As emphasized by Dr Daniel Clark, "Only, only, only Upper Cervical doctors have the ability to obtain that one thing: head-neck alignment—brain-to-body communication." [clxxxi]

━━━━━━━━━━━━━━

We have already discussed the vertebral arteries, which are the blood vessels that travel through the cervical vertebrae and supply blood to the cerebellum and the brainstem (See Chapter 7 and 8).

Certain chiropractic critics may argue that manipulation of the neck causes damage to these arteries, the consequence thereof being symptoms such as dizziness, nausea, headaches, slurred speech or blurry vision. These same individuals often raise additional concern that manipulation may even cause a cerebrovascular hemorrhage (i.e., stroke).

In response to such criticism and fear mongering, let me say first and foremost that chiropractic does not cause strokes. Medical and chiropractic expert Dr Scott Haldeman states that a stroke is a, "random and unpredictable complication of any neck movement including cervical manipulation," exceedingly rare and estimated to affect only 1 in 5.85 million people. [clxxxii]

Researchers have also noted that spinal manipulation imposes no elevated risk that a person may suffer a stroke compared to the general population. [clxxxiii]

It must be stressed that these findings are applicable only when treatment is administered by a licensed and proficient chiropractor. Would you ever have open-heart surgery performed by any person who is not a qualified cardiac surgeon? Of course not! That would be terribly risky!

Likewise, I would never recommend that you seek upper cervical treatment from anyone who is not an Upper Cervical chiropractor—especially if you have not had a proper examination and x-rays.

Alas, I have known many people who have visited so-called "atlas therapists" but have experienced strong adverse reactions following treatment. As it turned out, these therapists were not Upper Cervical doctors, chiropractors, osteopaths or even physiotherapists.

In fact, many of these "atlas therapists" had no formal qualifications whatsoever!

It is my professional opinion that any "atlas treatment" performed by an unqualified therapist is as foolish as handing a child a loaded gun.

Upper Cervical care is a specialist discipline that requires intensive study, years of practice, and a willingness to discover new things along the way. I cannot emphasize it enough: only Upper Cervical chiropractors have the qualifications and skill to correct an atlas subluxation.

Anything less, now that is risky.

Upper Cervical Safety

To tell the complete story, Upper Cervical treatment does contains a small amount of risk even when performed by a qualified specialist.

In a retrospective study over the careers of 83 Upper Cervical chiropractors representing over 5 million treatments, it was found that approximately 31% of patients do experience at least one symptomatic reaction within 24 hours of treatment. [clxxxiv] [clxxxv]

The researchers noted the most common reactions were tiredness (10.4%), radiating pain (6.3%), neck pain (5.4%), dizziness (4.9%) and headache (4.2%), the vast majority of which being of mild intensity, short duration and having little impact on daily living. Intense symptomatic reactions were found to occur in only 5.1% of Upper Cervical patients. [clxxxvi]

However, of great importance, not one case of a stroke or permanent injury following an atlas correction was ever reported. [clxxxvii] In my own studies, I have never found a documented or even anecdotal case where an Upper Cervical specific procedure has been linked to a stroke or other serious injury.

A final important point of the aforementioned study is that 69% of Upper Cervical patients experience no adverse events at all. Moreover, when all patients were asked to rate their overall satisfaction with Upper Cervical care, the average score given was 9.1 with "10" being the best possible score. [clxxxviii]

Not a bad report card!

It should be clear that the benefits of Upper Cervical care far exceed any associated risks. Although treatment is not required for all people, I do advocate that people have their upper neck checked regularly: much like a dentist, once or twice per year to confirm that everything is still in good shape.

Case Report: Suboccipital Neuralgia

Jane had suffered suboccipital neuralgia for 15 years before she came to my office.

She described her pain as a "constant spasm ... like the entire back of my head is on fire." Jane described that the problem was so intense that she would suffer unrelenting, debilitating migraines for days at a time. Her only relief would come if she compressed and then stretched her upper neck. However, she added that any relief would last only 20 minutes.

What was worst, the problem caused her to wake every 30 minutes. Her longest night of uninterrupted sleep in the last 15 years was less than 3 hours!

Despite taking horse-strength painkillers, muscle relaxants and seeing numerous specialists over the years, nothing had helped her.

"You're my last hope," she said to me.

No pressure there!

When I examined the back of her neck, it was like pressing into a board. Considering the severity and chronicity of her condition, I informed her that her symptoms may intensify initially when I would adjust her.

She understood but agreed that it with was worth the chance.

I could feel that her suboccipital muscles relaxed immediately after the treatment. Jane also felt that something was different. In the first 24 hours, she described that she felt "giddy," like she wanted to burst out laughing for no reason.

Alas, over the next 24 hours, Jane's worst fears came true when her pain intensified. In my office with exhaustion on her face, tears in her eyes and desperation in her voice, she pleaded with me to help her. She was so afraid what would happen if we dared to perform a second adjustment.

Just as well. When I checked her, she was still holding her adjustment. We did not do anything on that visit.

I kept in contact with Jane's husband over the next few days, and he informed me that Jane was on the mend. However, he did not elaborate how she was doing.

Two weeks later I received a phone call from Jane. Straight away I could hear a major change in her voice: it was light, like the weight of the world had been lifted off her.

She explained that after she left my office, she had seen her specialist who gave her the same type of muscle relaxants that she had been prescribed many times previously. This time, however, the relaxants were having an effect.

Within a week and after she stopped taking the muscle relaxants, Jane described that the pain in her head had melted away to almost nothing. She could still feel pressure and tightness across the back of her head, but even then it was not nearly as severe.

Best of all, she said that she had slept 5 hours uninterrupted each night for the past week!

I told Jane how happy I was to hear this wonderful news. Despite the initial flare-up, Jane added that she was so pleased with the Upper Cervical treatment, which she realised after 15 long years allowed her body to start to mend itself.

Jane's experience serves as a reminder that all forms of healthcare including Upper Cervical contain some element of risk. Things do not always go as smoothly as we prefer. On the flip side, it also serves as a lesson that a symptomatic reaction may not only be a short-term transition as the body adjusts to the rapid changes.

As stated by Dr Daniel Kuhn, "You have to deal with that life power and respect it and work with it. Don't fight with it. Let it have its way. You can do that when you get rid of the cause of the interruption between the source and the body by correcting the Upper Cervical vertebral subluxation." [clxxxix]

All Things Take Time

I have said it several times that I do not have the power to heal anyone. Only your own body has that ability. My role is simply to remove nerve interference so that your body will work the way it is supposed to.

The length of time required for the healing process is extremely variable. Muscle memory, structural mal-adaptation and the amount of continual stress in your life are all huge factors that determine how quickly or how slowly your body can heal.

Many people who receive Upper Cervical care experience significant symptomatic improvements within 2-4 weeks of their first treatment.

However, the underlying neurological and structural changes that have occurred over time often take much longer to resolve.

For every year that you have had a subluxation uncorrected, it requires your body 1 month of continuous healing to undo the damage.

Imagine a 25 year-old woman tells you that she has been suffering intermittent headaches for two weeks. After asking a few questions, she remembers that she fell from a horse when she was 10 years old. She adds that her school teachers always used to comment on her "terrible posture." Although this woman's symptoms have been present for only a few days, her true problem has probably been present for over 15 years!

It comes as a surprise for many people when they discover the hard way that their problems will not disappear in a few days even though symptoms are relatively new. It comes as an even greater surprise when they learn that their underlying problem may take weeks or months to correct because they have ignored it for so long!

———————

There are no shortcuts with Upper Cervical care or with body healing. As amazing as it is when people need only one treatment to restore their life, these people tend to be exceptions rather than the rule.

For most people, healing is a process that takes time.

Admittedly, the better your overall state of health, usually the better your recovery will go. To undo the effects of muscle memory and structural mal-adaptation is like breaking a habit: it may take great effort initially, but it is achievable.

Rest assured that no matter how long your problem has been there and no matter how severe it is, you can still heal. Your body never forgets and never stops trying to heal itself.

All it requires is the time and opportunity to do so.

CHAPTER 19

The Adjustment Specific

*Courage is not the absence of fear, but the triumph
over it. The brave man is not he who does not feel
afraid, but he who conquers that fear.*

Nelson Mandela

It takes an experienced Upper Cervical doctor only a few minutes to complete a proper x-ray analysis. As a student, I was ecstatic to finish in about 15 minutes.

Just before I left Joe in Kevin and Rob's care, Louise had discovered a wheelchair.

"This should make your trip back upstairs much easier," she said to us.

Why didn't I think of that? Only a few days before I would receive the title "Doctor," and I still had so much more to learn!

Joe was resting again in his darkened room. I found my dad in his office chatting with Kevin. Also there was Rob, who was scrambling to jot a few notes on everything that we had done so far.

Poor Rob. It was hard enough for me, let alone a clinic rookie to keep track of everything that we had done that morning. How he ever assembled his final report, I have no idea.

"It's like you said," I reported to my dad, "His atlas is stuck on the right side, but he has a counter-rotation of C1 and C2."

I could see the strain on his face Dr Hannah double-checked my measurements. With a sigh he raised his head and stared straight at me as if to say, "What have I gotten myself into?"

What I learned from my dad in this defining moment was how a doctor must be brave in the face of adversity. With just four simple words, I learned how a doctor must take action despite fear in order to help another human being in need:

"Okay, let's try it."

With the decision made, my dad stood tall and led the three of us to Joe's room.

For Joe's sake we kept the lights off but left the door slightly ajar. A sliver of light was all that we would need anyway.

Dr Hannah had previously selected that we would perform the Upper Cervical treatment for Joe not by hand, but by using a table-mounted stylus instrument. The plan was that I would set the instrument to the angle that I had measured from Joe's x-rays; and then with just the click of a button, the instrument would produce a gentle wave-like force to correct the alignment of Joe's atlas.

After that, we would allow him to rest and see if there would be any change.

That was the plan at least.

"Because you're already lying there," my dad explained to Joe, "I'm going to check your legs to see if they are level. Then I'll have you sit up so I can feel the back of your neck."

"Okay," Joe replied.

Dr Hannah verified that Joe's legs were quite unlevel. Next he assisted Joe into a seated position to palpate his atlas. Even through the darkness I could see Joe wince as my dad pressed into the tight muscles and swollen nerves of his upper neck.

"It's pretty sore back there," Joe informed us.

Dr Hannah directed his attention toward me. "Can you setup the instrument?"

"Sure," I responded.

Even though I knew that the ultimate responsibility of this adjustment would lie with my dad, I felt that it was my x-ray setup, my analysis and thus my fault if anything bad happened to Joe.

"Joe," my dad explained, "All you have to do is lie down on your left side with your head resting on this headpiece. Jeffrey is adjusting the instrument to the angle we found on your x-rays. When you're ready, we'll bring it down so that the tip of the instrument touches the skin between your jaw and your ear. You probably won't even feel anything when we do the adjustment. Then I'll have you sit up to re-check you."

"Thank you," Joe said.

The clinic rules dictated that because Rob had not taken the Upper Cervical elective, he was not permitted to perform the treatment on his own. Although we had already bent so many clinic rules that morning), we were not keen to break any of them outright.

Fortunately, Dr Hannah had been through similar scenarios previously. My dad would place his finger atop the button, and then Rob would only have to press down on his hand to deliver the adjustment. Although absurd, this approach would ensure that Rob would receive proper credit for his entire role in the morning's events; and it would also ensure that everyone would be protected from a legal standpoint in case something bad happened.

"Are you ready, Joe."

"Yes."

As much as I wish I could say that I felt confident the treatment would work, I cannot. I was still filled with doubt. One after another, dozens of "What if?" questions raced through my head.

What if nothing happens?

What if he really is having a stroke?

What if he gets worse?

Dr Hannah assisted Joe onto his side and then delicately positioned his head and shoulders into the correct position for the treatment. No one in the room dared to breathe, let alone speak. My dad moved his finger toward the button.

With a simple nod, he directed Rob to push down on his hand. Click.

I have purposefully not stated which form of Upper Cervical treatment we used to treat Joe. If you read this book carefully, you will be able to figure it out from my description. However, I have chosen to be ambiguous on this detail for two important reasons.

First, I am confident that another Upper Cervical chiropractor could have used another method for Joe and would have achieved similar results.

Second, although I have ways of doing things in own practice, the purpose of this book is to share the knowledge of Upper Cervical in all its forms.

Key Differences

I have implied it several times throughout this book, but now I will state it clearly and unapologetically: Upper Cervical care is not the same as general chiropractic.

Foremost there is no sudden twisting or cracking of neck with Upper Cervical care.

General chiropractic requires that the neck be brought to the point of tension where the vertebra is stuck. Spinal manipulation then requires a practitioner to deliver an impulse beyond the vertebra's normal end range of motion in order to restore function.

To contrast, Upper Cervical care corrects the alignment of the atlas and the axis within their normal ranges of motion.

As I have stated previously, I have been a chiropractic patient all my life. I have no personal problems with spinal manipulation. However, I do have a problem with excessive manipulation.

In my own experience as a patient and doctor, I have found that excessive manipulation weakens the muscles and ligaments that provide spinal stability. As a direct consequence, people suffer joint hypermobility. If this happens, people are unable to hold their corrections long enough for their injuries to heal.

Think of it this way: if your body is hypermobile, it is just as easy to manipulate a vertebra into proper alignment as it is to knock it straight back out of alignment with even the slightest amount of stress. As a consequence, these people suffer recurrent sprain-strain injuries and require continuous therapy every few days just to keep their symptoms at bay.

Alternatively, the goal of Upper Cervical care is to allow the adjustment to hold for as long as possible: the fewer treatments, the better.

Case Report: Migraines

> Dana was a 20-year old university student, who suffered vicious migraines. After ten years of taking 8 - 10 strong painkillers per day, she had finally decided that enough was enough.
>
> She had also never visited a chiropractor before.
>
> "I'm a little scared about the whole neck cracking thing," she admitted.
>
> "Don't worry," I assured her, "I don't do it like th—"
>
> "Which is weird," she interrupted with a laugh, "because I crack my own neck all the time."

She then showed me exactly how she could do it. She tilted her neck to the side, and then quickly jerked her head in the opposite direction. I think I heard every joint from C2 to C7 click out of place!

"Sometimes it feels better, but sometimes it doesn't," she added.

I knew exactly what Dana was talking about because I used to do the same thing with my own neck. I also knew about the local endorphin release that you experience when you cavitate a joint this way.

Yes, self-manipulation can make you feel better for a little while. However, it can also cause instability, arthritis and the associated pain and injuries that go with it.

I explained to Dana the many reasons she should not crack her own neck. Number one, she was likely moving the vertebrae that were already hypermobile (i.e., moving too much), but not the one vertebra that actually needed to move.

Number two, she was likely making her primary subluxation worse every time she did it.

Number three, she was likely causing greater damage that would only make her headaches worse in the long term.

Dana's neck was a mess on x-ray. The normal lordotic curve in her neck was flipped backwards. Even at 20 years old she already had some evidence of degenerative arthritis in her lower neck.

I could also see that her head was sticking forward at least five centimetres. Remember that the head weighs 4.0 - 5.0 Kg, and that for every 2.5 cm of forward head carriage the weight of your head doubles. What I saw on Dana's x-ray meant that she was effectively carrying a 16 - 20 Kg bowling ball on her shoulders every day.

No wonder she was suffering headaches!

I explained to Dana that I would not be cracking her neck, but instead that I would be performing a very specific correction. After the treatment, she was quite surprised.

"Well that didn't feel like anything at all."

"Just wait, and we'll see," I responded with a confident smile.

Sure enough, over the next two weeks Dana reported great improvements. On a scale from 1-10, she said that the intensity of her headaches dropped from "10" to a "2." She was having headaches only a couple of times per week, and she noted that she had not taken a single painkiller since her first treatment.

I was excited for Dana that Upper Cervical treatment was making such a profound difference for her already, but I knew that we still had a long way to go.

Three months later, Dana was still doing well and resisting the urge to crack her neck. Even when she gave into temptation, she noted that it would only click in one spot (which meant that her neck was stabilising).

Unfortunately, Dana was still suffering headaches every two weeks. That meant she was doing something that was preventing her adjustment from holding longer.

I ran through my usual list of questions: "Are you sleeping on your stomach, your side or your back? Are you sleeping with only one pillow? "Do you carry your school bag over both shoulders?" What about your purse? What about shopping bags?"

Eventually we discovered the problem. Dana was an avid fan of television crime drama. For a solid hour at least three times per week she would lie on a couch with her head propped awkwardly on the armrest.

"Well stop doing that and see what happens," I advised.

When I saw Dana two weeks later, she was fine. No headaches at all!

Over the next few weeks, we were able to reduce Dana's visits to once every 4 - 6 weeks. She also noticed that she could not physically crack her neck on her own. Or if she did, we would have about 24 - 48 hours to correct the problem or else she would suffer a migraine.

Not to be discouraged, Dana and I took this observation as a positive thing: it meant that Dana had an early sign that could help her to prevent her migraines by getting a re-adjustment before any symptoms would come.

That, I believe should be the ultimate goal of Upper Cervical care: to empower people to listen to their own bodies so that they know exactly what to do for themselves to get well and stay well.

———————

Another key difference between Upper Cervical and general chiropractic is that there is no cavitation, which is the cracking noise associated with spinal manipulation.

In defense of general chiropractic, there are a few important myths about joint cavitation that I would like to dispel. First, cavitation is not caused by bones rubbing against each other. The sound is nothing more than the sudden movement of fluid and air within a joint. It is the same type of sound produced when you pour milk into a bowl of cereal.

Second, joint cavitation by itself is usually completely harmless. It does not cause arthritis. It is only with excessive cracking (i.e., hypermobility) that degenerative arthritis may become a problem. It is one of the most important reasons I instruct people never to crack their own necks.

Third and probably the most important point from a chiropractic perspective, a cracking noise does not mean that an adjustment is always successful. Conversely, the absence of a cracking noise does not mean than an adjustment is unsuccessful either.

A one-gram cross-section of the trapezius (the broad muscle across the back of the neck and shoulders) contains 2.2 muscle spindles or sensors per gram of tissue. By comparison, the suboccipital muscles around the atlas contain between 100 and 250 spindles per gram. [cxc]

Recall that the atlas does not have any interlocking joints to hold it in place. It is suspended by these super-sensitive muscles and ligaments. Therefore, anything that stimulates your upper neck— even slight passive movements like when a chiropractor tilts your head to the side for a manual adjustment—causes the muscles to tighten... which keeps the atlas locked in place.

In my experience, I have found that cavitation associated with manipulation of the upper neck seldom comes from the atlas: instead, it comes from the joints of the lower neck.

I will testify that mobilization and manipulation of the upper neck absolutely provides effective symptomatic relief. I say it often, "There's a time when something's just gotta move." However, I will add that most of the time any such relief is short-term only.

General manipulation does not achieve the same type of correction that is provided with Upper Cervical care.

CHAPTER 20

The Atlas Correction

There is a power within
—a fountainhead of unlimited resources—
and he who controls it controls circumstances
instead of it controlling him.

Dr BJ Palmer

<hr>

The second law of Newtonian physics states that force is the product of mass and acceleration: F = ma. Considering that the suboccipital muscles are so sensitive, it should make sense that the most effective way to perform an Upper Cervical correction is to apply a very light impulse, but to do so extremely quickly.

The aim is not to use so much force that it hammers the atlas back into place. The secret of an Upper Cervical correction is to deliver a light force with such speed and precision that the atlas simply glides into its proper alignment on its own.

In order to prevent over-stimulation of the suboccipital muscles, the treatment requires that a patient's head lays on a supportive headpiece. In this manner, Upper Cervical chiropractors do not hold (or twist) the neck at all during the procedure.

Depending on the technique used by the doctor, the force of the treatment may be applied by hand or with instrument. The doctor places a hand or instrument onto the patient's neck, and then simply directs a vectored impulse through the plane of the atlas.

With rotational problems, the doctor does not twist the patient's neck, but simply torques the hand in an appropriate clockwise or counterclockwise direction.

That's it!

For the outside observer, Upper Cervical adjusting methods and instruments sometimes look a little strange. However, if you have ever experienced a treatment yourself, you would know that the procedures are quite safe, extremely gentle and also extremely effective.

The Sensation of Healing

Many people do not notice any immediate changes following an Upper Cervical correction. If you are suffering severe pain and take a painkiller, you usually don't feel instantly better either.

True healing takes time.

Although it is not as common, some people do feel a little worse following treatment. I never like it when people say they feel worse.

However, I know that it is sometimes a necessary step in the healing process.

For example, you may experience a stronger headache when your brain suddenly receives a normal amount of blood flow if it has been receiving only a trickle for so long. Or you may feel a whole body ache when your muscles suddenly start functioning again after years of inactivity.

There is also the phenomenon known as retracing, which occurs commonly in Upper Cervical practice.

Let's assume that you suffered an injury A. As a result of injury A, you suffer a series of progressive, related problems over a period of time: first B, then C, and now finally D.

Whether these problems are physical, chemical or emotional, as your body starts to heal itself, it retraces or goes backwards through the same sequence of problems in reverse order.

In other words, you may again experience the symptoms associated with D then C then B before finally arriving back at A before the original injury.

In the above cases, these symptoms (however unpleasant) are normal sensations as your body returns to normal

Fortunately, it has been my experience that most people notice positive, if not dramatic improvements following an Upper Cervical correction.

Some people comment that they feel so tired and relaxed that they could immediately fall asleep. Some people say it is like someone has removed a grainy film from their eyes and that they can see clearer. Others say it is like someone has cleared the fog from inside their head and that they can think better.

Other people I have known have experienced giddiness, gassiness, uncontrollable laughter or goose bumps following treatment. Others yet have described "warm" or pleasurable waves that have coursed through their bodies from head to toe.

My own mother reports that she feels a "lifting" sensation on the top of her head and a bit of lightheadedness following a successful treatment.

A sensation of lightheadedness—i.e., your neck feels looser and that your head feels lighter—is very common following an Upper Cervical treatment.

For these and any other changes that you may experience following treatment, all are positive indicators that the procedure is having a positive effect on your body.

Upper Cervical Methods

As described previously, there are six major forms of Upper Cervical treatment:

- Toggle Recoil (aka HIO or Palmer Upper Cervical Specific),
- Kale (aka Upper Cervical Knee Chest Specific),
- Blair,
- Orthospinology (aka Grostic),
- NUCCA and
- Atlas Orthogonal (AO).

Why do these different methods exist? The short answer is professional opinion and preference. Like all people, Upper Cervical chiropractors have their own opinions and experiences of what constitutes "the best" adjustment. The same is true among medical doctors, dentists and surgeons as well.

If I may critique my own profession, chiropractors are overly defensive when it comes to our treatment methods. What we forget is that most people do not care what the treatment is as long as it works!

When questions arise on the effectiveness of chiropractic and Upper Cervical care, my answer is simple: all forms of chiropractic work well to resolve chiropractic problems ... but for Upper Cervical problems, Upper Cervical care works best.

When it comes to Upper Cervical methods, no single approach is dominant to the others. They all achieve life-changing results.

The original HIO procedure used a knee-chest style table where patients would kneel on a small table and rest their heads sideways on an elevated headpiece. The Upper Cervical doctor would then deliver a high-velocity, low amplitude (HVLA) thrust to correct the vertebral subluxation without twisting or cracking the neck.

The closest living relative of HIO is the Kale method, which has maintained the original style and knee-chest style table. Despite its orthodoxy, Kale remains at the forefront for research, education and public awareness for Upper Cervical care.

Most other Upper Cervical methods have come to favour a side-lying table where the patient lies on his or her side. Two of these methods are Toggle Recoil and the Blair procedure. Both methods use an HVLA thrust with torque to adjust the atlas and the axis. A significant difference from the Kale method is that they use a drop mechanism incorporated into the headpiece.

Kale, Toggle Recoil and Blair generate 14.5 – 17.3 Kg of thrusting force to correct an atlas subluxation. [cxci] With the drop mechanism, however, the amount of force physically felt by the patient is far less than that. In fact, many people scarcely report feeling any pressure at all. In this manner, Toggle and Blair are extremely gentle even though they do generate more force than other Upper Cervical methods.

Kale, Toggle Recoil and Blair are classified as articular techniques. All three operate on the premise that the upper vertebrae should be in neutral alignment with the foramen magnum, which is the large opening in the skull where the brainstem sits. In particular, the Blair method emphasizes how congenital anomalies and joint asymmetries affect the ability of an Upper Cervical chiropractor to correct an atlas subluxation.

On the other side are the orthogonal techniques: Orthospinology, NUCCA and AO. These methods operate with the theoretical ideal that the upper cervical vertebrae should be perpendicular or at right angles with the spinal cord itself.

Although these three techniques focus on C1 and C2, treatment is limited to the atlas. The correction of an axis subluxation is achieved by adjusting the atlas against the axis and by using the leverage of a stationary headpiece and the patient's shoulder positioning.

As opposed to using an HVLA thrust to adjust the atlas, Orthospinology and NUCCA doctors apply a controlled downward pressure followed by a sudden release, which achieves the exact same results. The amount of force is usually 4.0 Kg, which is approximately the same that a patient would feel with a Toggle Recoil or Blair treatment. [cxcii]

Unlike the aforementioned techniques, Atlas Orthogonal is not performed by hand at all. Instead, AO uses a solenoid instrument, which creates a percussive wave-like force to adjust the atlas. It is similar to a Newton's Cradle (Figure 20.1). Because the impulse is much faster by machine than by hand, Atlas Orthogonal is often regarded as the lightest of all Upper Cervical methods.

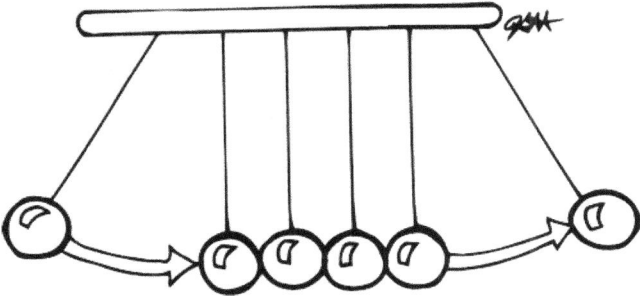

Figure 20.1. The Transfer of Force to Correct the Atlas

Case Report: Emily's Story (Part III)

> In truth, I had no idea if Emily's condition would improve.

> Would it take two weeks or two years? Would it happen suddenly or gradually? Would it happen at all?

"What I'll recommend is that we take things on a day-to-day basis over the next month." I explained to Christine and Emily. "Worst-case scenario, there will be no change. But if there is a change, then we you can decide how you'd like to take it from there."

Despite having so many of Emily's x-rays, MRIs and other scans on my desk, I did not have a single picture of her upper neck in a neutral position. I needed a proper set of Upper Cervical x-rays before I could adjust Emily.

With the first picture I could see part of Emily's problem clearly. Not only was her neck curve reversed from normal, but her atlas, which should have been angled 30 degrees upward, was angled 5 degrees downward!

Emily's neck would usually respond well. The muscle tension and discomfort she felt through her neck and spine would dissipate within a few moments after treatment. I imagined that her atlas was like a release-valve mechanism. If I could release the tension at one end of her spine, it would be easier to release the tension at the opposite end.

Then when both the atlas and the sacrum would be free to move, the rest of her spine should be able to unravel itself. Again, that was my hypothesis.

I worked with Emily almost every day for two full weeks. In the beginning, her adjustment would hold for only 24 hours before her muscles pulled everything back out of alignment. Toward the end of the second week, her adjustments were holding almost 48 hours.

Seeing Christine and Emily on a daily basis, I developed a special rapport with them. During this time, Christine would give me one of the nicest compliments I could have received.

"For all the specialists we've seen, you're the first one who didn't just say, 'There's nothing that can be done.' And you're the only one who's actually taken the time to explain things. Even if there's no change with Emily, thank you for trying."

Her words reminded me of a lesson my dad had repeated many times when I was a child and also when I was a student at Palmer.

"What is the only thing worse than failing?" he would ask. " ... Not trying."

Despite the compliment, I was feeling a bit disheartened that nothing appeared to be happening for Emily. She was still wheelchair-bound, and her body was as twisted and rigid as ever. I had no idea that I was about to see an exceptional change when Christine and Emily would next come to my office.

"She's not wearing her brace today," Christine explained. "It hurts more when I wear the stupid thing," Emily added with contempt. "Plus my back cracked last night."

"She took it off so that she could do the stretches you gave her," Christine continued. "While she was doing them I heard her back go 'click.' It wasn't the same as the loud 'pop' that was on the video, but it was the first time I've heard her back make any noise in months. Is that okay? Should we be doing that?"

Yes! I thought to myself. The tension is finally releasing.

"In her case," I responded, "I think that's okay."

I explained that the click in Emily's back was a sign that her body was retracing and that her joints were starting to unlock. It also meant that we were finally making real progress.

There is hope!

For all the wonderful news that Emily and Christine shared that day, it was what happened the next day that was beyond my wildest expectations.

(Concluded in Chapter 23)

━━━━━━━━━━━━━━━

When a joint is really locked up, spinal manipulation is a very appropriate form of treatment. General chiropractic can provide rapid relief for many symptoms including headaches and neck pain. However, if it is an upper cervical problem that has caused that joint to become stuck in the first place, then any symptomatic relief will be short-lived so long as the primary subluxation remains.

As described by Dr Julie Mayer Hunt, "You can adjust a low back problem all that you want, but if that weight of the head is still off centre, the minute [you're] standing up in a gravitational field, you're going to go back into the same pattern." [cxciii]

It is true that any significant stress may cause a subluxation to relapse. However, when the atlas is allowed to heal within its normal range of motion, it often stays put better with Upper Cervical care than any other form of treatment.

As Dr Drew Hall describes it: "It's holding the adjustment that gets people better. It's not adjusting them. It's keeping the interference checked out over a period of time that allows people to heal and repair and get back to a normal state of health." [cxciv]

CHAPTER 21

Health and Healing

Chiropractic is healthcare. Premiums small, dividends large.

Dr BJ Palmer

Dr Daniel Clark describes the healing process:

"Health and healing messages leave the brain by way of the brain stem, pass through the neck, down the spinal cord, out over the entire nervous system to all parts of the body. These messages control everything that goes on in the body. These messages also direct all body healing.

"Head-neck misalignment can cause interference at the point where the head and neck join and prevent the brain from sending its healing messages to the body.

"We know the brain controls everything that goes on in the body. So if the brain can't communicate with some part of the body, it's going to get sick. But if the brain can communicate with all parts of the body, we stay well." [cxcv]

High blood pressure. Sleeping disorders. Seizures. Nocturnal enuresis (bed wetting). Vertigo. Migraines. Sciatica. Jaw disorders. Asthma. Fibromyalgia. Multiple Sclerosis. Ear infections.

These are not problems that just happen to people for no reason. Every effect has a cause, and every cause effects. Moreover, it is possible that one cause may have thousands of potential effects.

There are thousands of medical conditions or diagnoses. However if a person has an atlas subluxation, there is but one cause and thus one solution.

However strong these statements, I do not mean to imply that Upper Cervical care is the panacea, the one-and-only cure for all health conditions in the known universe.

Many Upper Cervical chiropractors treat only the upper neck and achieve excellent results. However, Upper Cervical care often has its greatest impact working in conjunction with other forms of healthcare.

Although it is easy to forget, Upper Cervical chiropractors are doctors first, chiropractors second, and Upper Cervical practitioners third. As a doctor first, my primary duty is always to ensure that my patients receive the most-appropriate healthcare that is available to them.

Therefore, if a person does not have an Upper Cervical problem, has a dangerous condition, or does not experience any improvements after 2-4 weeks of treatment, then it behooves me to seek the expertise of other healthcare specialists.

Ultimately, it is about patient care. It is about your needs and your goals. And it is about you taking control of your life so that you can feel your best for as long as possible.

Your Habits Determine Your Life

Imagine that you have driven the same car for the past ten years. You have had the car serviced exactly as recommended by the manufacturer, and you have never been involved in an accident. Even if you have travelled less than 100,000 km in that time, it is still highly unlikely that your car drives just as brilliantly as the day you bought it.

Your body is a biomechanical machine similar to this car in many ways. Even though things may not work quite as well as they did when you were 16 years old, if you use your body properly (i.e., you exercise it), give it the best fuel (nutrition), take it for regular maintenance (chiropractic), and never get into a major accident, it will stay in good condition for a long time.

On the other hand, if you abuse your body, eat rubbish, and suffer various injuries along the way without ever seeking professional help, your body will rust, ache and break down well before you reach your 50th birthday.

The first important difference between your body and a machine is that a machine does not have self-healing abilities. If your body was not able to heal itself, you would probably suffer breakdowns every time that you worked too long, slept too little or lifted too much. Although your body is able to adapt to stress for chronic periods, there is still only so much stress that your body can handle before it snaps.

There is a second important difference to consider between your body and a car: you do not have the option to trade-in your old body for a new one even if you completely wreck it.

There is no way to guarantee that you will be perfectly healthy and injury-free for 100 years or longer. However, common sense and sage advice go a long way:

- Eat nutritious food including lots of fresh fruits and vegetables;
- Drink lots of pure water;
- Enjoy regular cardiovascular exercise;
- Get adequate amounts of sleep every night; and
- Be true to yourself, set your own goals and live according to your own standards.

Alas, many people ignore common sense, make poor choices, suffer lives of scarcity, and expect health providers to give them their health in the form of a tiny pill.

Albert Einstein said, "Insanity is doing the same thing over and over again and expecting different results." Insanity is also the false belief that you can have a healthy life without doing anything to achieve it.

Health is a direct reflection of your values and your habits.

_____

Simple but Not Always Easy

The healing process may be difficult for people for many reasons. However, there are two delicate but important things that people need to consider before commencing care: resources (i.e., money), and commitment.

On the first issue, people may not have the time or means to afford the treatment they require. However, the solution often boils down to a matter of priorities.

It never ceases to amaze me how people spend so much time, money and energy on things like houses, cars, gadgets and toys, yet how little they spend on things that will maintain their health.

In truth, Upper Cervical care is far from expensive—especially if you consider the cost of things like dentistry, surgery and the yearly cost of medical prescriptions ... not to mention the intangible pain and suffering that goes with delaying treatment.

The sad part is that many people do not make health a priority until it is already lost. Sadder yet, the cost to repair a problem that has been put-off for years is always greater than the cost it would have been to prevent it from happening in the first place.

Always remember that there is not a drug or exercise in the world that can fix an atlas subluxation.

_____

The second issue may be even more delicate. Simply put, many people do not want to do what it takes to get well. Again, the solution often boils down to a matter of priorities.

Do you really want to get well? If so, what are you willing to do to achieve it?

Many people expect to find health inside a little bottle (and then say that remembering to take it 3x a day is too hard)! Remember from previous chapters that all forms of stress—whether physical, chemical or emotional—have the same effect on your body. Therefore, it is usually some stressful element of your lifestyle that is preventing you from achieving the health that you desire.

It may be the stress of driving to work everyday.
It may be the stress associated with your diet.
It may be the stress of not having enough money.
It may be the stress associated with the nature of your work.
It may be the stress of a relationship that you can't seem to escape.

To overcome these types of problems, I believe the saying is true that, "The solution is simple but not always easy." It requires tremendous willpower to change these types of things.

That is the very reason why so many people struggle with their health.

Of course, I do not know what situations you face in your own life. Whatever it may be, I hope sincerely that you seek to overcome your challenges in order to discover the health and happiness that you deserve.

To achieve the life that you desire requires a change in values, a change in thought, and then a deliberate change of action. It requires that you to take proper care of your body. It requires that you engage in activities that will improve your health.

Fortunately, it does not have to be done all at once. I advocate that it can be achieved one step at a time at a pace that is comfortable for you.

As the saying goes, "Everything you want in life is on the other side of fear." All you have to do then is take the first step.

Case Report: Vertigo

Nicole was a 40-year old mother of three, who was seeking help for a problem that had plagued her for over a decade.

"I started to experience random bouts of dizziness once a month or so. It wasn't serious and would go away in 30 seconds or less. At the same time I started to get ringing in my ears or 'tinnitus' as my doctor told me. She referred me to an EENT [ears, eyes, nose and throat specialist], who sent me for some tests including an MRI or my head. They couldn't find anything, but the EENT said it was probably Ménière's Disease.

"I had to research it on my own. I read that it can be caused by fluid or a viral infection of the inner ear. Is that right?"

"Yes and no," I informed Nicole. "From the medical perspective, Ménière's disease is said to be idiopathic, which means that they don't know what causes it. Saying that it is a virus is basically a default diagnosis when they can't find anything else.

"It's the same with fibromyalgia if you know anyone diagnosed with that. When a person suffers extreme fatigue, illness, heaviness and pain throughout the body for no apparent reason, doctors give a name to those symptoms. They call it chronic fatigue syndrome or fibromyalgia. But it isn't a condition or disease at all.

"Ménière's is the same. It is not a disease. It is the name of a syndrome given when a person suffers dizziness, tinnitus and vertigo for no apparent reason.

"However," I added to emphasise that Nicole should not abandon hope, "that is just one perspective. Ménière's can be caused by other things including a problem with the upper neck."

I asked Nicole to continue her story.

"I was able to manage it for 8 years, but two years ago I was in a minor car crash. Nothing serious, but a month later the vertigo started so strongly that I had to grab onto a table just to stay upright. This would usually happen 5-10 times per week for a couple minutes at a time. The worst one lasted a few hours. I had to lie on the floor until the room finally stopped spinning.

"The tinnitus also got much worse. I read that if you hold something to your ear like a seashell that you can drown out the ringing. I figured I'd give it a try and was surprised that it actually worked. Have you ever heard of that?"

"Honestly no," I replied, "but I'll never argue with anything that works."

"It really has," Nicole continued. "If I put on my headphones and listen to white noise for an hour the tinnitus goes away completely for a few weeks.

"But the dizziness, that's there all the time. The vertigo just comes without any warning, and I can never tell when it's going to happen. I've had to give up driving. My husband has to take me everywhere, but it's been so bad lately that I can't even go to the shopping centre."

For Nicole who could no longer leave the house without facing the real possibility of a serious attack, the fear she felt as her world was progressively shrinking around her must have been tremendous.

"I've been to all the chiropractors, naturopaths and Chinese medicine doctors in town, but none of them have been able to help. I went online and read about what you do with the atlas. I'm not expecting a miracle, and I know this might take some time to fix, but I decided it was worth a try."

Nicole lived 10 hours away and would only be in town for three days. With such little time, we started right away.

Nicole had a significant amount of rigidity through her neck and also a definite leg length inequality.   As I expected, her x-ray examination confirmed that her atlas was misaligned.

The physical changes after adjusting Nicole's upper neck were minimal at best. I checked her each of the next two days. Nicole was still experiencing dizziness, but on a positive note she had not suffered any vertigo. I advised Nicole to monitor her symptoms closely when she returned home.

I received a phone call one week later.

"Can I see you next week?" Nicole said. "I had a bit of vertigo yesterday, but that's been the only time since I first saw you. I haven't gone that long without it for two years!"

Nicole and her husband made the 20-hour round trip again. Even one week later, she still reported that was the only vertigo episode. I re-adjusted Nicole's atlas and again advised her to keep me updated with any changes.

The next time she called was a month later.

"Sorry I haven't called earlier. Life's been so busy. I wanted to let you know that everything is still good. I haven't had one bit of vertigo, and I can count the number of times I've had the dizziness on one hand since last time I saw you."

I would not see Nicole in person for another two months. Even then, the only thing that she mentioned was tightness along the base of her skull.

The best news was not how she was feeling: it was what she was doing. Nicole had driven herself to see me! Not only that, she had the confidence to walk outdoors, exercise and go out into public spaces without the fear that she would suffer an attack.

I am always delighted when people feel much better with Upper Cervical care. However, it is seeing them get their lives back on track that most touches me the most.

I had another patient, who suffered similar symptoms as Nicole. In his case, he could not wear a hat because even the light pressure of the headband was enough to trigger his headaches and dizzy spells. After working with him for a few weeks, he told me how happy he was just to wear a hat again!

Seeing Nicole with her life returned to her was seeing a different person who took nothing in life for granted. I continue to see her every few months just to make sure that everything continues to go well for her. Although she is not cured from all her Ménière's symptoms, the fact that she is able to enjoy her life again is just another testament to the life-changing possibilities that may unfold with Upper Cervical care.

CHAPTER 22

A Life of Your Own Choosing

*All processes in life take time. And with time comes
clarity and perspective at all levels: physical,
chemical and emotional.*

Dr Sarah Farrant

We've already identified three things that trigger symptoms: physical trauma, chemical imbalances and emotional disturbances. On the flip side, there are three necessary elements to maintaining your health:

- physical wellbeing;
- physiological wellbeing; and
- psychological wellbeing.

Physical Wellbeing

An Upper Cervical subluxation has the potential to create neural interference anywhere in the body. So too can any physical problem elsewhere in the body cause health issues.

Imagine that you are building a house. After planning there are two general stages in the building process. Stage 1 requires building a solid foundation: concrete, braces, struts, plumbing, wiring and other stuff like that. Stage 2 requires turning this shell of a building into a functional house: walls, floors, paint, appliances, water and electricity.

To build a healthy body requires the same two things: structure and function.

The majority of the people who visit my office have issues with the upper neck. However, many of them also have structural problems that are beyond my specialty.

- Spinal misalignments below the upper neck, in the pelvic or elsewhere in the body.
- Congenital problems such an anatomically short leg (known as anisomelia).
- Structural or arthritic conditions such as scoliosis or Ankylosing Spondylitis.
- Old injuries causing referred or phantom pain.
- Motor pattern imbalances: i.e., where a group of muscles that should contract in a certain order A-B-C-D are actually contracting A-D-B-C.

For these types of structural problems, here is where Upper Cervical care works best with general chiropractic, podiatry, orthodontistry, and orthopaedics.

The other side of physical wellbeing is proper body function.

Many people ask me if chiropractors and physiotherapists are some type of mortal enemies. In my opinion, the answer is "No." There is no conflict so long as both professions do what we are best at doing.

Upper Cervical treatment corrects problems associated with the structural part of the human body (joint alignment and nervous system integrity). Physiotherapy corrects problems associated with the functional part (muscle strength and stability).

For best results, the two should work together!

Beyond physical rehab, you have to use your body to maintain your health. In other words, you have to exercise. It does not mean that you have to run marathons or do 100 sit-ups every day (unless you really want to). What it does mean is that you need to engage in some form of weight-bearing activity that makes you break a sweat and gets your heart pumping for 15-30 minutes a day.

Exercise does not have to be serious, just regular. Or as Dr Mike Evans puts it, "Can you limit your sitting and sleeping to just 23 and a half hours per day?" [cxcvi]

Exercise keeps all parts of your body working properly. Not only does it minimize rusting (arthritis), osteoporosis and muscle wasting (called sarcopaenia), it also regulates your internal physiology, expels toxins, elevates your mood and calms your mind.

And yes, you may actually come to enjoy it too!

Upper Cervical care is a foundation for your physical wellbeing. However, you will achieve the best results when you pursue a fit and active lifestyle.

Physiological Wellbeing

Optimal health is not limited to physical wellbeing. It also requires physiological wellbeing, which refers to the nutrients, chemicals and substances that circulate through your body.

Every person in every part of the world knows it: you are what you eat. More appropriately, you are what your digestive tract absorbs. Thus, your health depends greatly on the nature of the building blocks that you put into your body.

Remember the story of the Three Little Pigs. The first pig builds a house of straw; the second pig builds a house of sticks; but the third pig builds a house of bricks. Only people who build their houses with brick (i.e., quality food) are able to stand against the forces within the world that may threaten their wellbeing.

There are approximately 72 essential nutrients required by the body. Proteins, carbohydrates and fats constitute the three types of macronutrients. Macronutrients are the building blocks and energy sources that the body requires to function, heal and repair itself.

In Australia and America where there are supermarkets in every town (and fast-food outlets on every street corner), macronutrients are in no short supply. Paradoxically, it is not the hyper-availability of food that causes the staggering rates of obesity in western societies. It is actually a deficiency of food.

Let me clarify: it is a deficiency of micronutrients that is the problem

Micronutrients include vitamins A, C, E, D, the complex of B vitamins, calcium, magnesium, potassium, and iron. Lesser known micronutrients also include vitamin H (biotin), vitamin P (hesperdin and citrus bioflavenoids), molybdenum, vanadium, choline and inositol.

Should you lack any one essential nutrient, your brain will shift your metabolism into protection mode. Even if you are morbidly obese, eating fewer than 1000 Calories (the energy derived from macronutrients) and exercising 5 hours per day, your brain will still believe that you are starving!

Until you supply your body with that one missing nutrient, you will not be able to shed an ounce of body mass.

You may be familiar with the term empty calories. Empty calories refers to any food or drink product that contains macronutrients but no micronutrients. Some common examples include white bread, beer, breakfast cereals and almost everything that you'll find packaged or shrink-wrapped in the supermarket.

Many of these food-like products are so highly processed that they have zero nutritional value (assuming they had any to start). Many commercial farming methods use synthetic chemicals that strip nutrients from the soil. The result is nutrient-deficient plants, fruits and vegetables.

To complicate matters, things such as alcohol, caffeine, cigarettes, pollutants, household chemicals and numerous medications deplete your body of its existing nutrient stores. Many food-like products also contain flavour substitutes, sweeteners, colours, preservatives and other additives that upset your body's metabolism. In sufficient quantities, they may even dampen or destroy your body's ability to heal and repair itself.

For the few micronutrients that do remain in your food, they may not be bioavailable. In other words, they may not be in a form that your body can readily absorb. For example, calcium is abundant in broccoli and milk. It is also abundant in rocks. However, your body can absorb calcium from only one of these three sources (despite what you may think, it isn't milk)!

As an important aside, plant-based foods are the most abundant sources of bioavailable vitamins and minerals. They provide almost all nutrients that you require to build and maintain a healthy body.

Micronutrient deficiencies are extremely common in western nations and may cause as many health problems as a vertebral subluxation: obesity, cancer, cardiovascular disease, chronic fatigue syndrome, osteoporosis, liver disease and bowel disorders just to name a few.

Nutrition is an immense subject far beyond the scope of this book. I recommend that you learn more from the experts in the field:

- *Changing Habits, Changing Lives,* by Cyndi O'Meara. [cxcvii]
- *The Omnivore's Dilemma,* and *In Defense of Food*, by Michael Pollan. [cxcviii]
- *Food Matters* (2008 Documentary). [cxcix]

The simplest nutritional advice that I have read comes from author Michael Pollan: "Eat food. Not too much. Mostly plants." [cc] To elaborate just a bit more, I advise the following:

- Quick-fix diets don't work. Choose sustainable eating habits instead.
- Drink water. Not coffee, not tea, not soft drink, not alcohol. Just water.
- Eat small portions throughout your day. You don't need much animal protein or grains. The majority of your nutrients should come from raw organic fruits, vegetables, legumes, nuts and seeds.
- Many over-the-counter supplement brands are useless. Seek the advice of a naturopath or nutritional expert before undertaking any dietary modifications.

Psychological Wellbeing

The third aspect of optimum health, psychological wellbeing is just as important as your physical and the former two.

Just as an electrical conduit that produces a magnetic field, your body also generates an energetic or biomorphic field. Research indicates that this field is greatly influenced by the thoughts that we hold in our minds.

Think of a computer. It has default settings and various software programs that load automatically when you start it. Good types of software may include things like word processors, games and web browsers. Basically, these are programs that allow you to use your computer properly.

On the other hand, you may also have bad types of software on your computer: spam programs, malware and viruses. When these things infect your computer, they will eventually cause it to slow, crash and die.

Similarly, there are default programs that operate within our brains. These programs form our beliefs, thoughts and emotions. Just as with computers, there are good and bad programs that dictate our actions, which ultimately shape our lives.

Remember that there is no disconnection between the mind and the body.

The placebo effect is the phenomenon whereby a person experiences healing from the belief alone that they will heal. Passion, gratitude, joy and hope all represent positive emotions, which have positive physiological effects that facilitate healing.

Conversely, the nocebo effect is the phenomenon whereby a person experiences illness or even death from the belief alone that they are sick. Depression, doubt, fear and anger represent negative emotions, which may damage the body as severely, if not more than physical trauma.

Any destructive habit such as an eating disorder or a gambling addiction may also lead the body to physical ruin.

As you may imagine, the solution for these types of problems is to reprogram your mind: reset your default settings, adopt positive ways of thinking and then change your behavioural patterns.

As I said in the beginning of this chapter, just because a solution is simple does not mean that it is easy. If you have battled addiction, experienced depression, or survived any major life tragedy, you would know exactly what I mean. However, you would also know that anything, no matter how ominous or impossible it may seem is achievable.

Never underestimate the power of your mind. If you have the desire, the focus and the discipline to pursue what you truly desire in life, you will achieve it.

———————

Whether it is universal energy, biomorphic fields, or the untapped potential of the human mind, medical science has not yet been able to measure these types of forces.

For this reason, natural healing, acupuncture and even Upper Cervical treatment are often difficult to study empirically. Basically, we observe that they work, but we can't demonstrate fully how they work.

Still there are countless amazing, if not miraculous stories of healing that defy explanation. Furthermore, an increasing number of scientific discoveries are supporting the theories that Upper Cervical chiropractors and natural healers have proclaimed for years.

A few resources that I strongly recommend on these subjects include the following:

- *The Biology of Belief,* by Bruce Lipton. [cci]
- *Evolve your Brain,* by Joe Dispenza. [ccii]
- *The Mind and the Brain,* by Jeffrey Schwartz and Sharon Begley. [cciii]

———————

That said, I believe firmly that the four critical elements to achieving optimum health are as follow:

- Regular cardiovascular exercise;
- Good dietary habits;
- Positive ways of thinking and habits; and
- Upper Cervical specific care (of course).

Many people seek quick-fix solutions for their associated lifestyle diseases. However, lifestyle diseases are brought about by lifestyle habits. The only way to improve a lifestyle disease is to make a lifestyle change.

Remember that for all the marvelous advances in medical science (and even Upper Cervical care), the power to heal comes from within you.

CHAPTER 23

Never Abandon Hope

Hope is the wellspring that feeds health and healing.

Dr Fred Barge

━━━━━━━━━━━━━━━━━━━

The brain controls all messages to every cell in the entire body, including messages of health and healing.

The upper cervical spine—the atlas and the axis—directly affects the spinal cord and the brainstem, which is the control centre of the brain.

If there is a misalignment of the upper cervical spine, the brain is not able to communicate properly with the rest of the body. As a direct consequence, health problems will begin to appear.

Upper Cervical is a specialist approach to chiropractic that corrects the misalignment of the atlas and axis, thereby restoring the health and optimal wellbeing of the body.

As I stated in the opening chapter, if you take nothing else from this book except this one message, I have accomplished my task.

If there is a second message that I would like to convey to you, it is a message of hope.

Dr Robert Brooks describes two approaches to healthcare.

"On the one side it says you're fundamentally flawed. You're going to have things go wrong with you during the course of your life that you're not going to recover from or get over. You're not smart enough to make your own decisions, so we need to be making them for you... This is called intervention.

"On the other side of that picture it says you come fundamentally perfect, and you have the ability to heal and recover from almost everything and adapt to anything you can't heal and recover from. [So] I'm going to empower you to make your own decisions because you're the only one who knows what's true to you ultimately. This is called non-interference.

"If I've got a cavity in a tooth, I need an intervention. But for health in general, I need to find out what's keeping my life from working and get that out of my life." [cciv]

By definition, an Upper Cervical correction is a type of intervention. However, its purpose is to restore your body to a state of non-interference so that you will be able to get well and stay well.

Case Report: Emily's Story (Part IV)

"What do you think you're doing?"

I tried to feign disapproval, but there was no way that I could conceal my delight. I'm sure Emily knew it as well when she decided to walk into my office on her own two feet that morning.

Christine was supporting most of Emily's weight, and she was still bent forward heavily and leaning to the side... but she was walking!

"It was last night," Christine started with tears in her eyes. "Emily was doing her stretches when she said that she wanted to try moving around. It was more of a shuffle than a walk, but she did it. I told her to take it easy, but at the same time I was just so happy to see her doing it."

Emily said very few words that morning. I suppose she didn't need to. Her dramatic entrance plus the bright glow on her face said far more than words ever could.

Although Christine and Emily had planned to return home in a couple of weeks, they decided to stay a little longer to see how much more Emily would be able to improve. We also wanted to stabilise her atlas so that she would not suffer a relapse as soon as she got home.

Over the next few weeks, Emily's transformation was absolutely incredible. Within a week of standing, she was walking on her own. Within a month, she was standing almost completely upright.

She also shared with me her plans to destroy her plastic spinal brace that she despised so much.

"When we get home I'm going to burn it," she said with devilish joy.

Even with so many positive changes, I could tell that Christine and Emily were longing to return home. Although she was far from cured, her atlas corrections were holding for two weeks at a time. Her body, now free of the interference that had nearly crippled her, would continue to heal itself, and she would continue to do better and better.

There were a few tears the morning they left for home, but it would not be the last time I would see them. Christine and Emily regularly visit during school holidays for a check-up just to be sure that everything is okay.

Trouble still seems to follow Emily—athletics, Oz Tag, skiing holidays, etc—but the most important thing is that her condition has never returned. I remember clearly during one visit where I checked Emily from head to toe.

"There's nothing for me to adjust today." I was able to state confidently. "There is nothing wrong with you. And if I didn't know better, I'd say there never was."

Over the next few years, Emily would go on to be one of the top students in her class. Not only would she receive top academic distinctions in her school, she would also receive several national awards for her musical achievements.

To summarise Emily's life since the day she learned to walk again, it has been filled with hope and abundance. How much of it she would have achieved otherwise, I'll never know.

Admittedly, I cannot say if it was Upper Cervical or SOT that was the most important element in Emily's recovery. Based on my experience working with her, I would estimate that 15% was SOT, 40% was Upper Cervical care, but 45% was Emily herself.

When faced with "incurable" ailments, many people abandon hope before they have explored all the possibilities. Neither Christine nor Emily ever abandoned hope. I believe that their spirit and sheer determination to find an answer for Emily's mysterious condition was the most important element, which brought her body back to life.

My role in her amazing transformation was minor. However, that is actually one of the best things about Upper Cervical care.

It is a small thing. It is a gentle thing. And it is also a simple thing.

However, when it is combined with energy and hope, it is one of the most powerful and life-changing things in healthcare.

When Nobody Can Help

For all the technological advancements of mankind, we scarcely understand anything about the life power that resides within each of us. Ayuverdic healing, traditional Chinese medicine, Native American shamanism, and other practices throughout history have all recognized that there is a vital unseen force that animates the living world.

Advances in quantum physics have suggested that there is a universal field or intelligence, which flows within each of us, unites us, and sustains the existence of all things. Moreover, the human mind appears to have an effect on this substance. In other words, our thoughts and emotions produce unconscious waves of vibration that act upon the ether of the universe to shape the very world that we perceive.

Alas, medical science has yet to acknowledge the full extent to which these forces influence our daily lives. They dismiss what they do not understand as myth, placebo or wishful thinking. In so doing, they condemn people to lives of misery and despair.

"There is nothing we can do to help you."
"Go home. You just have to live with it."
"We don't know what causes it, and there is no cure."
"Don't see a chiropractor—you might get hurt."
"Don't take supplements—you're wasting your money."

In my opinion, these types of phrases are the most damaging words in all healthcare. I would like to emphasize that no matter how severe, chronic or scary your condition may be, you do not have to live in a world of fear if you choose to live in a world of hope.

I am not talking about a charlatanistic, dangerous kind of hope. The hope that I am talking about is genuine hope for an empowered and fulfilling life.

As my dad would always respond when someone would say to him, "Nobody can help me."

"Thank goodness I'm a nobody."

CHAPTER 24

The Big Idea

Many patients imagine that they have tried every-
thing. True, they have used many remedies,
but they have never had
the cause of their infirmity adjusted.

DD Palmer

Upper Cervical care is the best kept secret in healthcare, but I hope that by writing this book that secret will be made known to everyone.

Just as I have shared my knowledge and experiences with you, so too do I hope that you share with your friends, family, or anyone else you believe may benefit from learning about Upper Cervical care.

It is the only way that things will ever change.

All things in life are possible: the only limitations are time and energy.

━━━━━━━━━━━━━━━━

As this book comes to its close, it is my sincerest hope that you may find your spirit renewed with the information and stories that you have read. If you have been suffering ill health, I hope this book has provided you some of the answers you have been seeking.

If you have never heard of or experienced Upper Cervical care, I hope you make use of your knowledge and take the next step. Again, it is the use of knowledge that is power.

Even if you do not find the answers you seek, I would still implore you never to abandon your hope. Your answer will be waiting for you to discover when you are ready.

As we return for the conclusion of Joe's story, I would like to share one final word from Dr BJ Palmer, which he called The Big Idea.

"A slip on the snowy sidewalk in winter is a small thing. It happens to millions. A fall from a ladder in the summer is a small thing. It also happens to millions.

"The slip or fall produces a subluxation. The subluxation is a small thing. The subluxation produces pressure on a nerve. That pressure is a small thing.

"That decreased flowing produces a dis-eased body and brain. That is a big thing to that man.

"Multiply that sick man by a thousand, and you control the physical and mental welfare of a city. "Multiply that man by one hundred and thirty million and you can forecast and prophesy the physical and mental status of a nation.

"So the slip or fall, the subluxation, pressure, flow of mental images and dis-ease are big enough to control the thoughts and actions of a nation.

"Now comes a man. Any one man is a small thing. This man gives an adjustment. The adjustment is a small thing.

"The adjustment replaces the subluxation. That is a small thing. The adjusted subluxation releases pressure upon nerves. That is a small thing.

"The released pressure restores health to a man. This is a big thing to that man.

"Multiply that well man by a thousand, and you step up the physical and mental welfare of a city. Multiply that well man by a million, and you increase the efficiency of a state. Multiply that well man by a hundred thirty million, and you have produced a healthy, wealthy, and better race for posterity.

"So, the adjustment of the subluxation to release pressure upon nerves, to restore mental impulse flow, to restore health, is big enough to rebuild the thoughts and actions of the world.

"The idea that knows the cause, that can correct the cause of disease, is one of the biggest ideas known. Without it, nations fall. With it, nations rise.

"This idea is the biggest I know of." [ccv]

A Life of Your Own Choosing

It was 11:30am by the time that we adjusted Joe. Although my lazy morning was completely gone, it had been well worth the effort.

Of the countless hours of study and clinical practice I endured during my years at Palmer, the lessons and memories of my final 90 minutes are the ones that I remember most vividly. It is also the experience that has had the greatest impact on my professional life.

There was only one more thing to do: wait and see if the treatment would have any effect.

The silence within the room was deafening. The click of the adjusting instrument still echoed through my ears. The only other sound I could hear was the thumping of my own heart.

Kevin, Rob and myself stood perfectly still as we waited for something, anything to happen. I stepped aside to give Dr Hannah ample room as he helped Joe rise slowly from his side and back into a seated position.

"Are you okay so far?" asked Dr Hannah.

Joe still had his eyes clenched firmly shut, and he was gripping hard onto the top of the adjusting table for support. I could tell he was afraid to open his eyes and suffer the devastating disappointment that his world would be spinning just as much as it was 60 seconds ago. I can only imagine what hopes and prayers raced through Joe's mind in that moment.

"So far so good," Joe replied.

My dad next palpated the back of Joe's neck to feel for any changes.

Click.

The sound was barely audible, but sharp enough that it caught all of us by surprise. Dr Hannah was pressing gently, but just that small amount of pressure must have been enough to allow the lower neck joints to release on their own.

"That doesn't normally happen," Dr Hannah said with a light smile.

I knew that a clicking sound was not a reliable indicator that an Upper Cervical correction had been successful. However, this sound was a sign that something in Joe's neck must have changed.

The adjustment had definitely done something, but I still had no idea what.

"It isn't as sore," Joe announced softly.

"That's good," my dad responded. He removed his hands from Joe's head and then stepped around to the front of the table.

"Joe, can you open your eyes?"

Joe hesitated but then slowly flickered open his eyes and blinked several times. Just as he was about to speak, he stopped.

Despite the dim light, I could see an expression of bewilderment on his face. He turned his head side-to-side a few times, rubbed his brow and blinked several more times. Again he tried to speak but no words came.

"What is it Joe?" my dad asked.

"... I can see you."

Now it was I who was lost for words. My racing heart skipped a beat, but for the first time in about three minutes I was able to take a breath.

Joe said it again. "I can see you. And its just one of you! It's still a little fuzzy around the edges, but I can see you clearly now."

"That's good Joe," my dad replied. Although he showed no sign of it, I'm sure he also felt great relief that Joe had not gotten worse after the treatment.

Still, Dr Hannah didn't want to be too optimistic just yet. "Let's just have you lie down and let that work in. Keep talking to me and tell me what you are feeling."

While Joe was lying on the table, my dad rechecked his leg length. Sure enough, Joe's legs were now perfectly level. Despite this objective sign, it was what Joe described in the next few minutes that was most incredible.

"My head feels light, like it isn't so heavy."

"It doesn't feel like the room is spinning."

"I don't feel sick anymore."

"I feel really tired, like I haven't slept in days."

"My headache is still there, but only a little bit behind my eyes."

"I don't know how to describe it, but my body just feels warm and better."

I can online imagine that it was like we were seeing someone wake from a coma. Small tears welled in the corners of Joe's eyes. Seeing his expression of pure joy and wonder on his face, it was then that I realised just how amazing the transformation that I had just witnessed was.

Kevin, who had enough faith in Upper Cervical that he brought Joe for treatment was overjoyed that his friend was going to be okay.

Rob, who had never before seen Upper Cervical in action was wide-eyed and speechless.

And I, who had studied Upper Cervical but had never experienced something so incredible, was utterly dumbfounded and awestruck.

I don't know why I did what I did next. Maybe I thought that Joe did not need another person hovering over him.

Maybe I thought that Dr Hannah still had many other patients to see that morning, and the longer that I stayed the harder it would be for him to get on with his day.

Maybe I thought that Rob would have a mountain of paperwork to complete and that I should get away from the clinic before I got roped into helping him (even though I had lost my lazy morning, there was still a whole afternoon to preserve).

In hindsight, I was probably experiencing some degree of shock. All I remember feeling was the pressing urge to leave.

"Well," I announced, "I think I'm going to get going."

My dad looked straight at me with sincere appreciation. "Thank you Jeffrey. I'll see you when I get home later."

And just like that, I turned and left the room.

It took 30 minutes of wandering around the Palmer campus that I finally snapped back into reality. I simply could not fathom the enormity of the events that had just transpired.

Did any of that just happen? How did that just happen? Was any of it real?

I also realised that I had never said goodbye to Joe.

How stupid!

I knew that I would head home soon. However I decided to swing through the clinic one last time to see if my dad needed any further assistance. In truth, it was just an excuse to see how Joe was faring.

Again, I slipped through the rear entrance of the clinic to avoid being seen without proper clinic attire. Despite it all, I still feared the disciplinary committee.

I arrived at my dad's office only to discover it empty.

He's probably with another patient. I thought. I guess I'll see Joe myself.

I started to head toward Joe's treatment room. However, it was by sheer luck that I saw them out of the corner of my eye.

I was so surprised that I could neither move nor speak. I could only watch from afar as Joe—a young man who only two hours earlier could not see straight, stand or even walk on his own—shook hands with my dad, turned, and then walked out of the clinic on his own two legs.

It was the first time I had ever seen the power of Upper Cervical care in action, and it remains one of the most inspiring sights I have ever seen in my life.

Epilogue

We never know how far reaching something we may think,
say or do today will affect the lives of millions tomorrow.

Dr BJ Palmer

───────────

Less than one week later I would graduate from Palmer. Two weeks after that I would board an airplane bound for Sydney, Australia.

For many years I had longed to travel there, but the first opportunity did not come until three months before I would meet Joe. Strange as it sounds, from the first day that I arrived, I knew that I was home.

To this day, I cannot explain it. It was not the sunshine, the surf, the girls or even the lifestyle. It was simply an inner sense that I was supposed to be here. I believe it as strongly today as I did then that I am meant to be here for some purpose.

What that purpose is I can only speculate.

For all my years of study, I expected to be a manual adjustor—never an Upper Cervical chiropractor. Growing up, I always depended on my dad to "fix me" whenever I injured myself or whenever I felt ill.

Spinal manipulation was the type of chiropractic that I had known all my life. However, in my final hours at Palmer, I would see a different side to chiropractic that I had never seen before and had never believed possible.

The events of that morning would re-play in my mind for many weeks.

Is there a reason that Joe was the last patient I saw at Palmer?

Is this the purpose, the reason that I feel compelled to go to Australia?

Is this what I am supposed to do with my life?

———————————

My first few months in Australia were hard for many reasons. I lived alone in a tiny flat no larger than an ordinary bedroom (that included the kitchen and bathroom area). I had no means of transport. Trips to the shopping centre were challenging enough, let alone trips to the beach or the city!

I will admit it also that I was also battling depression on a daily basis. Many days I would lose the fight. Somehow I still managed to keep pressing forward with the hope that my life would improve.

Eventually it would. Thanks to the Internet I still had my parents to guide me. I also had a small group of very special friends who helped me through some of the most difficult days of my life. For everyone whose sage advice helped me in those days, I am eternally grateful.

After months of soul searching, I would eventually discover an inner sense of peace. I knew that I could not be the chiropractor that I had long expected to be.

My passion was for Upper Cervical.

So that was exactly what I decided to do. Since then I have focused all my efforts into understanding the intricacies of Upper Cervical care and into using that power to help people get their lives back to normal.

For all the challenges, stressful days and nights, I can say with absolute certainty that it has been one of the best choices that I have made in my life.

———————————

Even half a world away, I still wondered how Joe was doing.

I still regretted that I did not see him off when he left the clinic that morning. Through various sources I did learn that Joe would improve steadily in the days following his treatment.

The question still remained: "How did such a terrible thing happen to such a young, healthy person?"

The answer would come with subsequent medical testing and MRI scans, which revealed a series of lesions within his brain and spinal cord. Joe was diagnosed with multiple sclerosis.

Terrible as any such diagnosis may be, there are two important points I would like to mention here.

The first point, Joe did not have a diagnosis when we treated him. His Upper Cervical treatment still worked! I have seen people told by their specialists that, "We don't know what's wrong with you, so there's nothing that we can do."

My point is that Upper Cervical care may still work even if no one has a name for the symptoms that you're experiencing!

The second and possibly more important point, Joe did not allow a diagnosis to ruin his life. Even while Joe was undergoing all his medical tests, he completed his chiropractic pre-requisite studies and started his first term at Palmer.

With these points in mind, if you have been dealing with some unknown or scary condition, I would like to leave you with this message.

It does not matter what symptoms, disease, diagnosis or condition that you have. If your atlas is properly aligned, your body will have the best chance to heal.

When the innate power and potential within your body is able to work without interference, anything is possible.

For any disease or diagnosis you may have, it does not define or limit who you are.

You can choose to live a life without fear. And it is my sincerest hope that you do.

Seven months later, I would have a short holiday overseas to visit my family. I arrived back in Davenport late on a Wednesday evening. Apparently, I needed some serious rest. For the first time since I was a teenager I slept until almost 11:00am!

My day started around lunchtime when I decided that a Palmer homecoming would be in good order.

I wandered the halls for an hour saying hello to the many friends, faculty and familiar faces that I had known over the years. I stopped in the bookstore to find some good-value deals but stayed there for another hour when I bumped into a classmate of mine. I next popped into the radiology department for another hour to visit Louise and the other blue coats.

"Have you met any nice girls yet?" It was a longstanding problem that as a student I studied so much (too much) that I never had much of a social life.

"Not yet, but I'm working on it." I answered a bit embarrassed.

Three hours of non-stop chatting plus the long flight the day before were starting to take their toll. I was overdue for an afternoon coffee.

As I was exiting a crowded hallway alongside the main clinic, I glanced to my right as a group of students walked past. It did not register with me initially, but as I snapped my head back, I recognized one person who stood frozen among the crowd staring right back at me.

It was the last person I thought I would ever see again.

The shock of recognition and expression in his eyes sent a tingling wave of goose bumps through spine. It took a moment to find my voice as I stepped forward to shake his hand for the first time.

"What are you doing here?"

"I'm going to take a neurophysiology test," Joe replied, shifting a stack of notes in his arms. "What are you doing here?"

"Just visiting for the day."

Joe called to his friends, who were hurrying up the staircase and whom I assumed were going for the same test. "I'll be right there!"

I realised that he would not be able to stay long, but even one minute was long enough to finally ask what I had wondered for several months.

"How have you been doing?"

"I've been doing great," he said with a bright smile. "A few challenges, but doing real well. I'm loving it here at Palmer and doing chiropractic. I just have to survive finals, but everything else is going great."

It was what Joe said next with small tears forming in the edges of his eyes that has stayed with me for many years since.

"Thank you, thank you... You helped save my life."

Humbled and speechless, I cannot remember exactly how I responded. As we shook hands farewell, he repeated, "I've got to go, but I didn't think I'd ever get to say it ... Thank you, thank you."

"It was a pleasure, Joe. Good luck."

After watching Joe run up the stairs to take his exam, I couldn't quite leave straight away. I stood motionless in the hallway reliving the events of that Monday morning. This time, however, I finally knew how that story would end.

BJ Palmer once said, "We never know how far reaching something we may think, say or do today will affect the lives of millions tomorrow."

I feel blessed that I have actually seen how such a small thing one day has made such a big difference the next.

Thank you, Joe.

About the Author

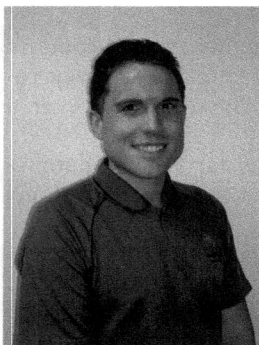

Dr Jeffrey Hannah is the principal Upper Cervical chiropractor with Atlas Health Australia. He is a graduate of Palmer College of Chiropractic in America, and he has worked in private practice for 5 years.

Jeff has previously been a chiropractic supervisor at Macquarie University in Sydney, and he still enjoys teaching and continues to work with students in Australia and abroad.

He has a special interest working with people, who have tried every other type of healthcare (including general chiropractic) but have not tried Upper Cervical.

Jeff and his wife Natalie are avid trail runners. They can usually be found on weekends (or weeknights) running somewhere in Brisbane Forest Park or the Sunshine Coast Hinterland.

References

Chapter 1

[i] What is Atlas Orthogonal? Sweat Institute for Atlas Orthogonal. 2010. http://www.sweatinstitute.com/content/whatsorthog.php.

[ii] Elert G. Mass of the Human Head. The Physics Factbook. Accessed 15 Dec 2011. http://hypertextbook.com/facts/2006/DmitriyGekhman.html.

[iii] Eriksen K. Upper Cervical Subluxation Complex: a review of the chiropractic and medical literature. Lippincott, Williams and Wilkins. Baltimore (MD). 2003:3-4.

[iv] Punjabi MM, White AA. Clinical Biomechanics of the Spine. JB Lippincott. Philadelphia (PA). 1978.

Chapter 2-3

[v] Farrant S. The Vital Truth: accessing the possibilities of unlimited health. JR Print. 2007:145-52.

[vi] What the Bleep do We Know!? Down the Rabbit Hole. Lord of the Wind Films. 2006.

[vii] Chudler EH. Dept Bioengineering, University of Washington (Seattle). 12 Oct 2010. Accessed 16 Aug 2011. http://faculty.washington.edu/chudler/ehc.html

[viii] Ibid.

[ix] What the Bleep do We Know!? Down the Rabbit Hole. Lord of the WindFilms. 2006.

[x] Feuling TJ. Chiropractic Works! Adjusting to a Higher Quality of Life. Wellness Solutions, 1999:150.

Chapter 4

[xi] Eriksen K. Upper Cervical Subluxation Complex: a review of the chiropractic and medical literature. Lippincott, Williams and Wilkins. Baltimore (MD). 2003:257-79.

[xii] Aprill C, Axinn MJ, Bogduk N. Occipital headaches stemming from the lateral atlanto-axial (C1-C2) joint. Cephalgia. 2002;22(1):15-22.

[xiii] Whittingham W, Ellis WB, Molyneux TP. The effect of manipulation (toggle recoil technique) for headaches with upper cervical joint dysfunction: a pilot study. J Manipulative Physiol Ther. 1994;17(6):369-75.

[xiv] Killinger LZ. A chiropractic case series of seven chronic headache patients. Palmer Res J. 1995;2(2):48-53.

[xv] Angus-Leppan H, Lambert GA, Michalicek J. Convergence of occipital nerve and superior sagittal sinus input in the cervical spinal cord of the cat. Cephalgia. 1997;17(6):625-30.

[xvi] Bovim G, Sand T. Cervicogenic headache, migraine without aura and tension-type headache: diagnostic blockage of greater occipital and supraorbital nerves. Pain. 1992;51(1):43-8.

[xvii] Bogduk N. The cervical-cranial connection. J Manipulative Physiol Ther. 1992;15(1):67-70.

[xviii] Eriksen K. Upper Cervical Subluxation Complex: a review of the chiropractic and medical literature. Lippincott, Williams and Wilkins. Baltimore (MD). 2003:327-30.

[xix] Hinson R, Brown S. Chiropractic management of trigeminal neuralgia: a preliminary study. 130th Annual Meeting of the American Public Health Association. 11 Nov 2002.

[xx] Weigel G, Casey KF. Striking back! The trigeminal neuralgia Handbook. Trigeminal neuralgia Association. 2000.

[xxi] Tomasi J. What TIME Tuesday? International Christian Servants, Inc. Broken Arrow (OK). 2005.

[xxii] Hinson R. Upper cervical neurology and trigeminal neuralgia. Abstracts from the 16th Annual Upper Cervical Spine Conference. 20-12 Nov 1999. Marietta (GA).

[xxiii] Knutson GA. Thermal asymmetry of the upper extremity in scalene anticus syndrome, leg-length inequality and rewponse to chiropractic adjustment. J Manipulative Physiol Ther. . 1997;20(7):476-81.

[xxiv] Glick DM. Conservative chiropractic care of cervicobrachialgia: a case study. Chiropr Res J. 1989;1(3):49-52.

[xxv] Eriksen K. Upper Cervical Subluxation Complex: a review of the chiropractic and medical literature. Lippincott, Williams and Wilkins. Baltimore (MD). 2003:243-56.

[xxvi] White B, Kessinger RC. The upper cervical spine and chronic lumbar disc degeneration with muscular atrophy. 17th Annual upper cervical spine conference. Life University. Marietta (GA) 3-4 Feb 2001. Chiropr Res J. 2000;7(2):82.

[xxvii] Kessinger RC, BonevaDV. The influence of upper cervical specific chiropractic care on lumbar range of motion. Abstracts from the 17th annual upper cervical spine conference. Life University. Marietta (GA). 3-4 Feb 2001. Chiropr Res J. 2000;7(2):80.

[xxviii] Dickholtz M, Woodfield C. Atlas correction of patients with neck and back pain using the NUCCA technique (abstracts from the 16th an-

nual upper cervical spine conference, 20-21 Nov 1999). Chiropr Res J. 1999;6(2):86-7.

[xxix] Pollard G, Ward G. The effect of upper cervical or sacroiliac manipulation on hip flexion range of motion. J Manipulative Physiol Ther. 1998;21(9):611-16.

[xxx] Robinson SS, Collins KF, Grostic JD. A retrospective study; patients with chronic low back pain managed with specific upper cervical adjustments. Chiropr Res J. 1993;2(4):10-6.

[xxxi] Eriksen K. Upper Cervical Subluxation Complex: a review of the chiropractic and medical literature. Lippincott, Williams and Wilkins. Baltimore (MD). 2003:376-85.

[xxxii] Kessinger RC, Boneva DV. A new approach to the upper cervical specific: part I. Chiropr Res J. 2000;7(1):14-32.

[xxxiii] Knutson GA. Rapid elimination of chronic back pain and suspected long- term postural distortion with upper cervical vectored manipulation: a novel hypothesis for chronic subluxation/joint dysfunction. Chiropr Res J. 1999;6(2):57-64.

Chapter 5

[xxxiv] The Power of Upper Cervical. Storyville Studios. 2007.

[xxxv] McAviney J, Schulz D, Bock R, Harrison DE, Holland B. Determining the relationship between cervical lordosis and neck complaints. J Manipulative Physiol Ther. 2005;28(3):187-93.

[xxxvi] Cailliet R. Neck and Arm Pain (2nd Ed). FA Davis. 1981.

[xxxvii] Eriksen K. Upper Cervical Subluxation Complex: a review of the chiropractic and medical literature. Lippincott, Williams and Wilkins. Baltimore (MD). 2003:386-88

[xxxviii] Ibid: 131-62.

[xxxix] Eriksen K. Correction of juvenile idiopathic scoliosis after primary upper cervical care: a case study. Chiropr Res J. 1996;3(3):25-33.

[xl] Travell JG, Simons DG. Myofascial pain and dysfunction: the trigger point manual. Volume 1. Baltimore, Williams and Wilkins. 1983.

Chapter 6

[xli] Cramer GD, Henderson C. Zygapophyseal joint adhesions after induced hypomobility. J Manipulative Physiol Ther. 2010; 33:508-18.

[xlii] Cramer GD, Fournier JT, Wolcott CC, Henderson NR. Degenerative changes following spinal fixation in a small animal model. J Manipulative Physiol Ther. 2004; 27: 121-154.

[xliii] Hoiriis K, Jordan J. Response of frozen shoulder syndrome to care by upper cervical chiropractic adjustments: a multiple case study. Conference

Proceedings of the Chiropractic Centennial Foundation. Washington (DC). July 1995;357-8.

[xliv] Feeley KM. Conservative chiropractic care of frozen shoulder syndrome: a case study. Chiropr Res J. 1992;2(2):31-7.

[xlv] Eriksen K. Upper Cervical Subluxation Complex: a review of the chiropractic and medical literature. Lippincott, Williams and Wilkins. Baltimore (MD). 2003:364-6.

[xlvi] Ibid: 362-4.

[xlvii] Eriksen K. Management of cervical disc herniation with upper cervical chiropractic care. J Manipulative Physiol Ther. 1998;21(1):51-6.

[xlviii] Robinson GK. Reabsorption of a herniated cervical disc following chiropractic treatment utilizing the atlas orthogonal technique: a case report. Abstracts from the 14th annual upper cervical spine conference, 22-23 Nov 1997. Life University. Marietta (GA). Chiropr Res J. 1998;5(1):41.

[xlix] Sweat RW. Correction of multiple herniated lumbar disc by chiropractic intervention. J Chiropr Case Reports. 1993;1(1):14-7.

[l] Eriksen K. Upper Cervical Subluxation Complex: a review of the chiropractic and medical literature. Lippincott, Williams and Wilkins. Baltimore (MD). 2003:334-7.

[li] Buskila D, Neumann L, Vaisberg G, Alkalay D, Wolfe F. Increased rates of fibromyalgia following cervical spine injury. Arthritis and Rheumatism 1997;40(3):446-52.

[lii] Woodfield C, Dickholtz M. the effect of upper cervical chiropractic corrections on patients with chronic fatigue syndrome. Abstract from the 15th Annual Upper Cervical Conference. 21-22 Nov 1998.

[liii] Amalu WC. Upper cervical management of primary fibromyalgia and chronic fatigue syndrome cases. Today's Chiropr. 2000;29(3):76-86.

[liv] What is a Subluxation? Upper Cervical Care: a new approach to healthcare. Upper Cervical Health Centers, Inc. DVD 2010.

[lv] A New Approach to Healthcare. Upper Cervical Care: a new approach to healthcare. Upper Cervical Health Centers, Inc. DVD 2010.

[lvi] The Power of Upper Cervical. Storyville Studios. 2007.

Chapter 7-8

[lvii] Lewellen GR. Human CNS Structure (5th Ed). Kendall/Hunt Publishing. Dubuque (IA). 2004:38-41.

[lviii] Schutte BL, Teese HM, Jamison JR. Chiropractic adjustments and esophoria: a retrospective study and theoretical discussion. J Aust Chiropr Assoc. 1989;19(4):126-8.

[lix] Gilman G, Bergstrand J. Visual recovery following chiropractic intervention. J Chiropr Res Clin Investigation. 1990;6(3):61-3.

lx   Terrett AGJ, Gorman RF. The eye, the cervical spine, and spinal manipulative therapy: a review of the literature. Chiopr Technique. 1995;7(2):43-54.

lxi   Kessinger R, Boneva D. Changes in visual acuity in patients receiving upper cervical specific chiropractic care. J Vertebral Subluxation Res 1998;2(1):43-9.

lxii   Eriksen K. Upper Cervical Subluxation Complex: a review of the chiropractic and medical literature. Lippincott, Williams and Wilkins. Baltimore (MD). 2003:339-44.

lxiii   Ibid: 364-6.

lxiv   James KA. Upper cervical chiropractic care for spasmodic torticollis cases: abstracts from the 15th annual upper cervical spine conference. 21-22 Nov 1998. Chiropr Res J. 1999;6(1):26.

lxv   Bolton PS, Bolton SP. Acute cervical torticollis and palmer upper cervical specific technique: a report on three cases. Chiropr J Aust. 1996;26(3):89-93.

lxvi   Killinger LZ. Torticollis: a chiropractic case study. Palmer Res J. 1995;2(2):23-6.

lxvii   Kaplan AS, Assael LA. Temporomandibular disorders, diagnosis and treatment. WB Saunders. 1991:456-460.

lxviii   Hannah DW. Iatrogenic trigeminal neuropathy with resultant atypical facial fasciculation of the zygomaticomandibularis: chiropractic and dental co-management. eJ Acad Chiropr Orthoped. 2007;4(1):4-10.

lxix   Kessinger R, Boneva D. Bell's palsy and the upper cervical spine. Chiropr Res J. 1999;6(2):47-55.

lxx   Hulse M. Cervicogenic hearing loss. HNO. 1994;42(1):604-13.

lxxi   Terrett AGJ. Vertebrogenic hearing deficit, the spine, and spinal manipulation therapy: a search to validate the D.D. Palmer/Harvey Lillard Experience. Chiropr J Aust. 2002;32(1):14-26.

lxxii   Eriksen K. Upper Cervical Subluxation Complex: a review of the chiropractic and medical literature. Lippincott, Williams and Wilkins. Baltimore (MD). 2003:345-6.

lxxiii   Ibid: 303-7.

lxxiv   Fallon JM. Chiropractic care of 401 children with otitis media: a pilot study. Alternative therapies. 1998;4(2):93.

lxxv   Burcon MT. Upper cervical protocol for ten meniere's patients. Ninth Annual Vertebral Subluxation Research Conference. 13-14 Oct 2001. Spartanburg (SC).

lxxvi   Boneva D. Two case studies: menieres disease and cervical spine trauma post upper cervical specific chiropractic care. Abstracts from the 15th Annual Upper Cervical Spine Conference. 21-22 Nov 1998. Chiropr Res J. 1999;6(1):24.

lxxvii   Heikkila H, Johansson M, Wenngren GI.   Effects of acupuncture, cervical manipulation and NSAID therapy on dizziness and impaired hear repositioning of suspected cervical origin: a pilot study. Man Ther. 2000;5(4):151-7.

[lxxviii] Eriksen K. Upper cervical subluxation complex: a review of the chiropractic and medical literature. Lippincott, Williams and Wilkins. Baltimore (MD). 2003:279-86.

[lxxix] Bakris G, Dickholtz M Sr, Meyer PM, Kravitz G, Avery E, Miller M, Brown J, Woodfield C, Bell B. Atlas vertebra realignment and achievement of arterial pressure goal in hypertensive patients. J Human Hypertension. 2007;21:347-52.

[lxxx] Hannah, JS. Changes in systolic and diastolic blood pressure for a hypotensive patient receiving upper cervical specific: a case report. Chiropr J Aust. 2009;39(3):118-21.

[lxxxi] Knutson GA. Significant changes in systolic blood pressure post vectored upper cervical adjustment vs control groups: a possible effect of the cervicosympathetic and/or pressor reflex. J Manipulative Physiol Ther. 2001;24(2):101-9.

[lxxxii] Nansel D, Jansen R, Cremata E, Dhami MS, Holley D. Effects of cervical adjustments on lateral-flexion passive end-range asymmetry and on blood pressure, heart rate and plasma catecholamine levels. J Manipulative Physiol Ther. 1991;14(8):450-6.

[lxxxiii] Tran TA, Kirby JD. The effects if upper cervical adjustment on the normal physiology of the heart. J Am Chiropr Assoc. 1977;14:59-62.

[lxxxiv] Eriksen K. Upper cervical subluxation complex: a review of the chiropractic and medical literature. Philadelphia (PA): Lippincott, Williams, and Wilkins; 2004:349-51.

[lxxxv] Purdy WR, Frank JJ, Oliver B. Suboccipital dermatomyotomic stimulation and digital blood flow. J Am Osteopathic Assoc. 1996;96(5):285-9.

[lxxxvi] Fujimoto T, Budgell B, Uchida S, Suzuki A, Meguro. Arterial tonometry in the measurement.of the effects on innocuous mechanical stimulation of the neck on heart rate and blood pressure. J Autonomic Nervous System. 1999;75(2-3):109-15.

[lxxxvii] Eriksen K. Upper Cervical Subluxation Complex: a review of the chiropractic and medical literature. Lippincott, Williams and Wilkins. Baltimore (MD). 2003:315-7.

[lxxxviii] Jackson R. The cervical syndrome (4th Ed). Charles C Thomas, 1977.

[lxxxix] Amalu WC. Chiropractic management of 47 asthma cases. Today's Chiropr. 2000;29(6):84-101.

[xc] Peet JB, Marko SK, Piekarczyk W. Chiropractic response in the pediatric patient with asthma: a pilot study. Chiropr Pediatrics. 1995;1(4):9-13.

[xci]   Kessinger R. Changes in pulmonary function associated with upper cervical specific chiropractic care. J Vertebral Subluxation Res. 1997;1(3):43-9.

[xcii]   Eriksen K. Upper Cervical Subluxation Complex: a review of the chiropractic and medical literature. Lippincott, Williams and Wilkins. Baltimore (MD). 2003:351-8.

[xciii]   Wiles MR. Observations on the effects of upper cervical manipulations on the electrogastrogram: a preliminary report. J Manipulative Physiol Ther. 1980;3(4):226-8.

[xciv]   Selano JL, Hihtower BC, Pfleger B, Collins KF, Grostic JD. The effects of specific upper cervical adjustments on the CD4 counts of HIV positive patients. Chiropr Res J. 1994;3(1):32-9.

[xcv]   Eriksen K. Upper Cervical Subluxation Complex: a review of the chiropractic and medical literature. Lippincott, Williams and Wilkins. Baltimore (MD). 2003:310-5,353-7.

[xcvi]   Ibid: 346-8.

[xcvii]   Carrick FR. Changes in brain function after manipulation of the cervical spine. J Manipulative Physiol Ther. 1997;20(8):529-45.

[xcviii]   Kelly DD, Murphy BA, Backhouse DP. Use of a mental rotation reaction- time paradigm to measure to the effects of upper cervical adjustments on cortical processing: a pilot study.   J Manipulative Physiol Ther. 2000;23(4):246-51.

[xcix]   Kessinger RC, Boneva DV. Neurocognitive function and the upper cervical spine. (Abstracts from the 16th Annual Upper Cervical Spine Conference, 20-21 Nov 1999). Chiropr Res J. 1999;6(2):88.

[c] Eriks Eriksen K. Upper Cervical Subluxation Complex: a review of the chiropractic and medical literature. Lippincott, Williams and Wilkins. Baltimore (MD). 2003:318-9.

[ci]Pistolese RA. Epilepsy and seizure disorders: a review of literature relative to chiropractic care of children. J Manipulative Physiol Ther. 2001;24(3)199-205.

[cii]   Eriksen K. Upper Cervical Subluxation Complex: a review of the chiropractic and medical literature. Lippincott, Williams and Wilkins. Baltimore (MD). 2003:319-21.

[ciii]   Pistolese RA. Epilepsy and seizure disorders: a review of literature relative to chiropractic care of children.   J Manipulative Physiol Ther. 2001;24(3):1999-205

[civ]   Amalu WC. Cortical blindness, cerebral palsy, epilepsy and recurring otitis media: a case study in chiropractic management. Today's Chiropr. 1998;27(3):16-25.

[cv]   Elster EL. Upper cervical chiropractic management of a patient with parkinson's disease: a case report.   J Manipulative Physiol Ther. 2000;23(8):2000.

cvi   Elster EL. Upper cervical chiropractic management of a multiple sclerosis patient: a case report. J Vertebral Subluxation Res. 2001;4(2):22-30.

cvii   Killinger LZ, Azad A. Multiple sclerosis patients under chiropractic care: a retrospective study. Palmer Res J. 1997;2(4):96-100.

cviii   Kirby SL. A case study: the effects of chiropractic on multiple sclerosis. Chiropr Res J. 1994;3(1):7-12.

cix   Eriksen K. Upper Cervical Subluxation Complex: a review of the chiropractic and medical literature. Lippincott, Williams and Wilkins. Baltimore (MD). 2003:404-5.

cx   Ibid: 291-5.

cxi   Goodman RJ. Attention deficit disorder (ADD) and the atlas subluxation complex. Upper Cervical Monograph. 1994;5(4):17-8.

cxii   Eriksen K. Upper Cervical Subluxation Complex: a review of the chiropractic and medical literature. Lippincott, Williams and Wilkins. Baltimore (MD). 2003:318-26,397-400.

cxiii   Elster EL. Upper cervical chiropractic care for a nine-year-old male with tourette syndrome, attention deficit hyperactivity disorder, depression, asthma, insomnia, and headaches: a case report. J Vertebral Subluxation Res. Jul 2003:1-11.

cxiv   Thomas MD, Wood J. Upper cervical adjustments may improve mental function. J Man Med. 1992;6:215-6.

cxv   Aguilar AL, Grostic JD, Pfleger B. Chiropractic care and behavior in autistic children. J Clin Chiropr Pediatr. 2000;5(1):293-304.

Chapter 9

cxvi   The Power of Upper Cervical. Storyville Studios. 2007.

cxvii   Ibid.

cxviii   Palmer DD. The Science, Art and Philosophy of Chiropractic. Portland Printing House. Portland (OR). 1910.

cxix   Daniel David Palmer. Wikipedia. Accessed 27 Feb 2012. http://en.wikipedia.org/wiki/Daniel_David_Palmer#cite_note-textbook-1.

cxx   BJ Palmer. Wikipedia. Accessed 27 Feb 2012. http://en.wikipedia.org/wiki/B.J._Palmer

cxxi   The History of Chiropractic. Wikipedia. Accessed 27 Feb 2012. http://en.wikipedia.org/wiki/History_of_chiropractic

cxxii   Palmer BJ. Hole-In-One therapy Absolutely Right. Fountainhead News. 1930;18(3).

cxxiii   BJ Palmer. Wikipedia. Accessed 27 Feb 2012. http://en.wikipedia.org/wiki/B.J._Palmer

Chapter 10

[cxxiv] Eriksen K, Rochester RP. Orthospinology Procedures: an evidence-based approach to spinal care. Lippincott, Williams and Wilkins. Philadelphia (PA). 2007;14-5.

[cxxv] Palmer BJ. The Subluxation Specific-The Adjustment Specific. Palmer School of Chiropractic. Davenport (IA). 1934.

[cxxvi] Eriksen K, Rochester RP. Orthospinology Procedures: an evidence-based approach to spinal care. Lippincott, Williams and Wilkins. Philadelphia (PA). 2007;18-24.

[cxxvii] Society of Chiropractic Orthospinology. www.orthospinology.org.

[cxxviii] NUCCA: National Upper Cervical Chiropractic Association. www.NUCCA.org.

[cxxix] Atlas Orthogonality. www.atlasorthogonality.com

[cxxx] Advanced Orthogonal. www.advanedorthogonal.com.

[cxxxi] Upper Cervical Specific Chiropractic: Kale World Headquarters. www. kale.org.

[cxxxii] Blair Chiropractic Society. www.blair.org.

Chapter 11

[cxxxiii] Chapman CD. Stress and the Subluxated Spine—with some "Lite" Thermodynamics. Upper Cervical Monograph. 1999;6(1):7-9.

[cxxxiv] Eriksen K. Upper cervical subluxation complex: a review of the chiropractic and medical literature. Lippincott, Williams and Wilkins. Baltimore (MD). 2003:37.

[cxxxv] What is Body Imbalance? Upper Cervical Care: a new approach to healthcare. Upper Cervical Health Centers, Inc. DVD 2010

[cxxxvi] What is Upper Cervical Care? Ibid.

[cxxxvii] O'Neill. Obstetrics and Pediatrics. Brady Press. Davenport (IA). 2007:72-3.

[cxxxviii] Seidel HM, Ball JW, Dains JE, Benedict GW. Mosby's Guide to Physical Examination (5th Ed). Mosby, Inc. St Louis (MO). 2003:945-8.

[cxxxix] Eriksen K. Upper Cervical Subluxation Complex: a review of the chiropractic and medical literature. Lippincott, Williams and Wilkins. Baltimore (MD). 2003:300-3.

[cxl] Gutmann G. Blocked atlantal nerve syndrome in infants and small children. Manuelle Medzin, Springer-Veriag. 1987. (As published in ICA International Review of Chiropractic. 1990;46(4):37-43.

Chapter 12-13

[cxli] Krafft M, Kullgren A, Lie A, Tingval C. Assessment of Whiplash Protection in Rear Impacts. Swedish National Road Administration & Folk-

sam. April 2005. Accessed 6 Oct 2011. http://web.archive.org/web/20070808142807/.

cxlii Sapountzi-Krepia DS, Valavanis J, Panteleakis GP, Zangana DT, Vlachojiannis PC, Sapkas GS. Perceptions of body image, happiness and satisfaction in adolescents wearing a Boston brace for scoliosis treatment. J Adv Nurs. 2001;35(5):683-90.

cxliii Marchiori D. Clinical Imaging with Skeletal, Chest and Abdomen Pattern Differentials. 2nd Ed. Elsevier Mosby. St Louis (MO). 2005:956.

cxliv Eriksen K. Upper Cervical Subluxation Complex: a review of the chiropractic and medical literature. Lippincott, Williams and Wilkins. Baltimore (MD). 2003:287-99.

cxlv Wiberg JM, Nordsteen J, Nilsson N. The short-term effect of spinal manipulation in the treatment of infantile colic: a randomized controlled clinical trial with a blind observer. J Manipulative Physiol Ther. 1999;22(8):517-21.

cxlvi Klougart N, Nilsson N, Jacobsen J.Infantile colic treated by chiropractors: a prospective study of 316 cases. J Manipulative Physiol Ther. 1989;12(4):281-8.

cxlvii Butler S. Headaches a real pain-in-the neck. Telegraph. 27 Aug 1970: 27.

Chapter 14-15

cxlviii What is Body Imbalance? Upper Cervical Care: a new approach to healthcare. Upper Cervical Health Centers, Inc. DVD 2010.

cxlix Rochester RP, Owens EF. Patient placement error in rotation and its affect on the upper cervical measuring system. Chiropr Res J. 1996;3(2):40-53.

cl Harrison DE. Repeatability over time of posture radiograph positioning and radiograph line drawing: an analysis of six control groups. J Manipulative Physiol Ther. 2003;26(2):87-98.

cli Jackson BL, et al. Reliability of the pettibon patient position system for radiographic production. J Vertebral Subluxation Res. 2000;4(1):3-11.

clii Rochester RP. Inter and intra-examiner reliability of the upper cervical x-ray marking system: a third and expanded look. Chiropr Res J. 1994;3(1):23-31.

cliii Eriksen K, Owens EF. Upper cervical post x-ray reduction and its relationship to symptomatic improvement and spinal stability. Chiropr Res J. 1997;4(1):10-7.

cliv Eriksen K. Upper cervical subluxation complex: a review of the chiropractic and medical literature. Lippincott, Williams and Wilkins. Baltimore (MD). 2003:16.

clv Anderson RT. A radiographic test of upper cervical chiropractic theory. J Manipulative Physiol Ther. 1981;4(3):129-33.

clvi Eriksen K, Rochester RP. Orthospinology Procedures: an evidence-based approach to spinal care. Lippincott, Williams and Wilkins. Philadelphia (PA). 2007;20.

clvii Eriksen K. Upper cervical subluxation complex: a review of the chiropractic and medical literature. Lippincott, Williams and Wilkins. Baltimore (MD). 2003:83.

clviii Ibid.

clix A New Approach to Healthcare. Upper Cervical Care: a new approach to healthcare. Upper Cervical Health Centers, Inc. DVD 2010.

Chapter 16

clx Eriksen K. Comparison between upper cervical x-ray listing and technique analyses utilizing a computerized database. Chiropr Res J. 1996;3(2):13-24.

clxi Ibid.

clxii Eriksen K. Upper cervical subluxation complex a review of the chiropractic and medical literature. Lippincott, Williams and Wilkins. Baltimore (MD). 2003:184.

clxiii A cubic millimeter of your brain. The Astronomist. 27 Jul 2011. Accessed 28 Sept 2011. http://theastronomist.fieldofscience.com

clxiv Information about radiation dose for patients. Queensland X-ray. Accessed 27 Sept 2011. Sunnybank (Q). 2010 http://www.qldxray.com.au

clxv Radiation Exposure in X-Ray and CT Examinations. Radiological Society of North America. 14 July 2011. Accessed 28 Sept 2011. http://www.radiologyinfo.org

clxvi Ibid.

clxvii Information about radiation dose for patients. Queensland X-ray. Accessed 27 Sept 2011. Sunnybank (Q). 2010 http://www.qldxray.com.au

clxviii Ibid.

clxix Ibid.

clxx Ionising Radiation and Health. Australian Radiation Safety and Nuclear Protection Agency. 25 Mar 2011. Accessed 28 Sept 2011. www.arpansa. gov.au/radiationprotection

clxxi Hannah JS. Upper cervical chiropractic treatment for a patient demonstrating a non-traumatic bipartite atlas: a literature review and case report. Chiropr J Australia. 2009;39(2): 70-4.

Chapter 17

clxxii Eriksen K. Upper Cervical Subluxation Complex: a review of the chiropractic and medical literature. Lippincott, Williams and Wilkins. Baltimore (MD). 2003:189.

clxxiii Ibid. 131-62.

clxxiv   Ibid. 208.

clxxv   Palmer BJ. Fountain Head News. (1924);14(3):15.

clxxvi   Palmer T, Denton K, Palmer J. A clinical investigation into upper-cervical biomechanical stability: part I. Upper Cervical Monograph. 1990;4(10):2-7.

clxxvii   Uematsu S, Edwin DH, Jankel WR, Kozikowski J,   Trattner M. Quantification of thermal asymmetry: Part 1. Normal values and repro-ducibility. J Neurosurg 1988;69:552-5.

clxxviii   Seemann DC. Anatometer measurements: a field study intra- and inter-examiner reliability and pre to post changes following an atlas adjustment. Chiropr Res J. 1999;6(1):7-9.

clxxix   Lawrence D. Lateralization of weight in the presence of structural short leg: a preliminary report. J Manipulative Physiol Ther. 1984;7(2):105-8.

clxxx   Ibid.

Chapter 18

clxxxi   The Power of Upper Cervical. Storyville Studios. 2007.

clxxxii   Haldeman S, Kohlbeck FJ, McGregor M. Risk Factors and Precipi-tating Neck Movements Causing Vertebrobasilar Artery Dissection After Cervical Trauma and Spinal Manipulation. Spine. 1999;24(8):785-94.

clxxxiii   Cassidy JD, Boyle E, Côté P, He Y, Hogg-Johnson S, Silver FL, Bondy SJ. Risk of vertebrobasilar stroke and chiropractic care: results of a population-based case-control and case-crossover study. Spine. 2008;33:176-83.

clxxxiv   Eriksen K, Rochester RP, Hurwitz EL. Symptomatic reactions, clini-cal outcomes and patient satisfaction associated with upper cervical chiropractic care: a prospective, multicenter, cohort study. BMC Musculoskele-tal Disorders. 2011. http://www.biomedcentral. com/1471-2474/12/219

clxxxv   Leboeuf-Yde C, Hennius B, Rudberg E, Leufvenmark P, Thunman M. Side effects of chiropractic treatment: a prospective study. J Manipulative Physiol Ther. 1997;20(8):511-5.

clxxxvi   Eriksen K, Rochester RP, Hurwitz EL. Symptomatic reactions, clini-cal outcomes and patient satisfaction associated with upper cervical chiropractic care: a prospective, multicenter, cohort study. BMC Musculoskele-tal Disorders. 2011. http://www.biomedcentral.com/1471-2474/12/219

clxxxvii   Ibid.

clxxxviii   Ibid.

clxxxix   Brain to Body Communication. Upper Cervical Care: a new approach to healthcare. Upper Cervical Health Centers, Inc. DVD 2010.

Chapter 19-20

[cxc] Kulkarni V, Chandy MJ, Babu KS. Quantitative study of muscle spindles in suboccipital muscles of human foetuses. Neurol India. 2001;49(4):355-9.

[cxci] Sweat RW. Atlas orthogonal percussion adjusting instruments. Today's Chiropr. 1984;13(3):31-3.

[cxcii] Grostic JD. The adjusting instrument as a research tool. Chiropr Res J. 1988;1(2):47-55.

[cxciii] A New Approach to Healhcare. Upper Cervical Care: a new approach to healthcare. Upper Cervical Health Centers, Inc. DVD 2010.

[cxciv] The Power of Upper Cervical. Storyville Studios. 2007.

Chapter 21-24

[cxcv] The Power of Upper Cervical. Storyville Studios. 2007.

[cxcvi] Evans M. 23 ½ Hours - What is the Single Thing We Can Do for Our Health. Accessed 30 Mar 2012. www.youtube.com/watch?feature=player_embedded&v=aUaInS6HIGo

[cxcvii] O'Meara C. Changing Habits, Changing Lives. Penguin Books. 2000.

[cxcviii] Pollan M. In Defense of Food: an eater 's manifesto. Penguin Books. 2008.

[cxcix] Food Matters. Permacology Productions. 2008. www.foodmatters.tv.

[cc] Pollan M. In Defense of Food: an eater 's manifesto. Penguin Books. 2008.

[cci] Lipton B. The Biology of Belief: unleashing the power of consciousness, matter and miracles. Hay House. 2005.

[ccii] Dispenza J. Evolve Your Brain: the science of changing your mind. Health Communications. 2007.

[cciii] Schwartz J, Begley S. The Mind and the Brain: neuroplasticity and the power of mental force. RegenBooks. 2002.

[cciv] The Power of Upper Cervical. Storyville Studios. 2007.

[ccv] Palmer BJ. The Big Idea. Rondberg TA. Chiropractic First. The Chiropractic Journal. 1996:130-1.